30% off PTCB Hero Online!

Thank you for buying **PTCB Hero: The Essential Information You Need to Pass the First Time (and Nothing Else!)**. We know you'll pass your PTCE with flying colors once you've absorbed all the information in this short, fluff-free guide.

Do you want to cement your knowledge and make sure you *really* understand it? Do you wish to feel reassured that you can recall that knowledge under exam conditions – with the types of questions that will appear on the real thing?

Then look no further than **PTCB Hero Online** – the perfect complement to this book. When you buy **PTCB Hero Online**, you'll get:

- **Hundreds of practice questions** with complete explanations of the correct answers (you can focus on one knowledge domain at a time, or mix them up)

- **Two simulated exam**s with complete explanations of the correct answers

- **A condensed version of this book** – so you can learn on your device whenever you have a spare moment

PTCB Hero Online is compatible with computers, smartphones, and tablets, so you can access it whichever way you please.

Visit www.ptcbhero.co and enter 30OFFNOW at checkout for 30% off.

If you have any questions or concerns before you buy, simply email admin@medicalhero.co and we'll get back to you right away!

PTCB Hero:

The Essential Information You Need to Pass the First Time (and Nothing Else!)

2021–2022

By the Medical Hero Team

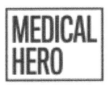

Contents

About This Book

PTCB Hero: The Essential Information You Need to Pass the First Time (and Nothing Else!) is different from your regular PTCB exam study guide. Why? Because we haven't filled it with lots of unnecessary information – the type of information that'll take forever to learn and NEVER be on the exam. Instead, it contains only the information that's essential for passing. Nothing else!

In order to pass, however, we don't believe it's enough simply to read the information and hope for the best. You need to study in a way that suits you, in order to make sure you're able to retain the information and recall it at the key moment: during the exam itself. That's why the first section of this book outlines some tactics for figuring out your learning style, making the most of your study sessions, and approaching exam day fully prepared.

(It's also a good idea to put your new knowledge to the test with some online practice tests and simulated exams. Ours are the best when it comes to how realistic they are! Head to **www.ptcbhero.co** to see what's included, then enter **30OFFNOW** at checkout for 30% off.)

There's some other information about the PTCB exam and the role of the pharmacy technician near the front of the book – just in case you need it. The rest of the book is devoted to teaching you the essential information for each PTCB knowledge domain.

Who are we?

Medical Hero (the creators of PTCB Hero) consists of a team of medical test prep experts who know what it takes to succeed the first time. Our study materials are consistently kept up-to-date, and they include everything you need to pass your written exams. We want to make test prep fast, efficient, and effective – and we're rooting for you to succeed in becoming a certified pharmacy technician.

We have a number of PTCB specialists on the team, but our lead experts are HaVy Ngo, Pharm.D. and Patricia Weiser, Pharm.D.

> HaVy Ngo graduated from Auburn University Harrison School of Pharmacy with a Doctor of Pharmacy (Pharm.D.) degree. With experience in both hospital and community pharmacy settings, Dr. Ngo is passionate about guiding patients to better health through medication therapy and lifestyle counseling. She is certified in sterile compounding. Dr. Ngo is working on a Master of Business Administration degree with a concentration in Healthcare Management from Mercer University in Atlanta.

> Patricia Weiser, Pharm.D., is a graduate of the University of Pittsburgh and a licensed community pharmacist. She is also an experienced health content writer and consultant. Before Patricia became a pharmacist, she was a nationally certified pharmacy technician.

A quick note about the URLs used in this book

There are a few website links scattered throughout this book. Rather than giving you the original – often ridiculously long – link, we've chosen to create shorter ones that are easier for you to type, but will take you to the exact same page.

Here's an example: to link you to a page from the U.S. Bureau of Labor Statistics about pharmacy technician earnings, you'll see that we provide you with this URL later in the book: **www.ptcbhero.co/earnings**. The original URL is **https://www.bls.gov/ooh/healthcare/pharmacy-technicians.htm#tab-5**, but we think ours is easier to type! Both URLs will take you to the same page, but we only include the shorter, easier one in this book. (Be sure to type the full link into the search bar of your browser – don't search for it in Google as it won't work that way!)

Let's get started!

Now that you know all about this book and why we created it, it's time to get started on the rest of it. Let's go!

Short Glossary

CPhT: Certified Pharmacy Technician. This is the official name for the role you wish to be certified for. Throughout this book you'll see that references to "CPhT" and "pharmacy technician" are used interchangeably. Please note, however, that in other settings, "pharmacy technician" can also mean non-certified pharmacy technicians: not all states require their pharmacy technicians to pass a certification exam. (Some states simply ask that their pharmacy technicians be licensed or registered, whereas others don't even require licensing or registration – let alone exam certification. There's more on this later in the book.)

PTCB: Pharmacy Technician Certification Board. PTCB is one of only two organizations in the country to offer CPhT certification. Out of the two, the PTCB certification is the only one that's accepted in every U.S. state and territory.

PTCE: Pharmacy Technician Certification Exam. This is the exam provided by PTCB, which you must take in order to become a certified pharmacy technician. In this book "PTCE," "PTCB exam," and simply "exam" are all used interchangeably.

Understanding the Role of a Pharmacy Technician

What Does a Pharmacy Technician Do?

A pharmacy technician is different from a pharmacist. While pharmacists have different responsibilities and expertise, pharmacy technicians still have an extremely important job to perform – one that requires diligence, math and organizational skills, attention to detail, and a friendly and helpful manner. Their role is to be a valuable and helpful assistant to the pharmacist – and indeed, pharmacists rely on pharmacy technicians and would not be able to do their job without them.

Pharmacy technicians work in many different settings, including hospitals, long-term care facilities, and – most frequently – retail pharmacies. In 2019, 51% of pharmacy technicians worked in pharmacies and drug stores, 17% worked in hospitals (state, local, and private), and 9% worked in food and beverage stores. (Source: www.ptcbhero.co/jobsettings.)

Depending on the state, a pharmacy technician may do the following:

- Measure, mix, compound, and fill bottles with prescribed medications, and label them with directions and other relevant information for patients (under the supervision of a pharmacist)

- Answer the phone and greet people entering the store

- Contact doctors' offices to confirm dosing instructions (or to confirm their approval or request prescription renewals)

- Process payments using the cash register

- Resolve issues and complaints with customers

- Keep detailed records of on-hand medications and other stock

- Deal with any issues concerning patients' insurance coverage

So what does that leave for the pharmacist to do? Their job involves reviewing and approving all medication orders before they're dispensed, preventing harmful drug interactions from occurring, managing the pharmacy technician team, and administering or supervising vaccinations. A pharmacist also has ultimate responsibility at the pharmacy – for their own work, their technicians' work, and for the overall professionalism of the pharmacy's operations.

Note: a key difference between both roles (**which you must know for your exam**) is that the pharmacist can legally counsel patients on the safe and appropriate use of their medication. They may also offer advice to doctors regarding the type and dosage to prescribe. A pharmacy technician is not allowed to do this.

Due to the differences in the nature of the work, the level of education required for each job differs considerably – although both require plenty of hard work, dedication, and learning. The requirements to become a pharmacy technician will be explained shortly.

What Are the Job Prospects for Pharmacy Technicians?

According to the Bureau of Labor and Statistics (BLS), employment of pharmacy technicians is expected to grow 4% between 2019 and 2029. (Source: www.ptcbhero.co/outlook.)

According to the BLS, this projected growth is based on a number of factors:

- The population is aging, and older people "typically use more prescription medicines than younger people."

- Increasingly higher rates of chronic diseases (such as diabetes) among all age groups will lead to an increased demand for prescription medications.

- "Advances in pharmaceutical research will allow for more prescription medications to be used to fight diseases."

- Pharmacy technicians will be needed to "take on a greater role in pharmacy operations because pharmacists are increasingly performing more patient care activities, such as giving flu shots. Technicians will need to perform tasks – such as collecting patient information, preparing more types of medications, and verifying the work of other technicians – that were previously done by pharmacists."

In contrast, the BLS predicts that employment of pharmacists will *decline* by 3% over the same period – partly because "fewer of these workers are expected to be needed as pharmacy technicians increasingly perform tasks previously done by pharmacists, such as collecting patient information, preparing some types of medications, and verifying the work of other technicians." (Source: www.ptcbhero.co/outlookpharma.)

Despite the excellent job prospects for pharmacy technicians, there is still competition: there are many applicants for each pharmacy technician role. How can you stand apart from the rest and get the job?

How to stand out from the other job candidates

Not all states require you to pass a certification exam in order to become a pharmacy technician. But if you live in a state where exam certification *isn't* required, passing a certification exam tends to make it much easier to distinguish yourself from other candidates and get a job. For more information about certification, read the chapter called "What Is PTCB Certification?"

There's more you can do too, however, to stand out from other pharmacy technician candidates:

1. Gain experience in customer service (and inform the pharmacy you're applying to about this experience). Pharmacy technicians spend a lot of time interacting with customers, so it's a good idea to practice!
2. In your interview, be sure to mention that you're proficient at performing pharmacy-related calculations.
3. You'll have to balance many responsibilities as a pharmacy technician. Ensure your résumé provides examples of occasions when you've had to be incredibly organized.

So... obtain your PTCB certification, then show evidence of your skills in customer service, math, and organization, and you'll be on your way to your dream pharmacy technician job!

But what can you expect to earn once you're employed?

How much do pharmacy technicians earn?

According to the BLS, the median annual wage for pharmacy technicians was $35,100 in May 2020. The highest 10% of pharmacy technicians earned more than $50,430. (Source: www.ptcbhero.co/earnings.)

Pharmacy technicians working in hospitals (state, local, and private) earn the highest median annual wages:

- Hospitals (state, local, and private): $39,290 (median annual wage)

- Pharmacies and drug stores: $33,110 (median annual wage)

- Food and beverage stores: $32,320 (median annual wage)

Pharmacy technicians working in other settings earned a lower median wage than the ones listed here.

What are examples of future job opportunities for pharmacy technicians?

Once you have some experience as a pharmacy technician, you can choose to specialize in a number of areas or move to a different kind of career within the medical field – all of which are more advanced than entry-level positions and may come with a sizeable salary increase.

Some examples are:

- Lead pharmacy technician

- Pharmacy affairs program manager

- Pharmacy technician instructor/educator

- Oncology pharmacy technician

- Nuclear pharmacy technician

- Institutional pharmacy technician

- Pharmacy purchasing agent

- Medication reconciliation technician

- Managed care pharmacy technician

- Pharmaceutical sales representative

- … And many more

Understanding PTCB

What Is PTCB Certification?

In order to become a pharmacy technician, many states require that you become licensed or registered first. Sometimes, this licensing/registration involves simply having a high school diploma and completing on-the-job training, but in many states you also need to become certified by passing an exam. (Very few states require no sort of licensing, registration, or certification.) To find out the specific requirements in your state, visit www.ptcbhero.co/states.

As we mentioned earlier, if you live in a state where exam certification is *not* required, we recommend you take a certification exam anyway and become a Certified Pharmacy Technician (CPhT). Passing the exam is a simple way to distinguish yourself from other candidates and prove you have all the knowledge required to be an excellent pharmacy technician – and as a result, you'll probably find it much easier to get a job.

Two organizations offer certification: the Pharmacy Technician Certification Board (PTCB) and the National Healthcareer Association (NHA).

PTCB is the nation's first and most trusted pharmacy technician credentialing organization, which is why pharmacy technicians with a PTCB certification in particular have a better experience when looking for a job (and being promoted once in the job). Employers recognize that, through the PTCB credentialing program, PTCB-Certified Pharmacy Technicians will have all the qualifications, knowledge, and experience necessary to perform the duties of a pharmacy technician. What's more, PTCB is the only pharmacy technician certification accepted in every U.S. state and territory.

Once you become a Certified Pharmacy Technician through PTCB, you can advance your career through other PTCB certifications as well as assessment-based certificate programs:

Certifications (of which the CPhT is one) "assess an individual's mastery of job knowledge, require Continuing Education, and award an acronym after one's name." One such certification is the Compounded Sterile Preparation Technician Certification (CSPT) – which "provides the opportunity to be recognised by your employer and colleagues for successfully meeting PTCB's rigorous requirements for this advanced credential."

There is also the Advanced Certified Pharmacy Technician Certification (CPhT-Adv), which recognizes "expertise and experience," and demonstrates "an unwavering commitment to advancing medication safety." Active CPhTs who have "completed at least four assessment-based certificate programs including Technician Product Verification Certificate (TPV) and/or Medication History, or three certificate programs and PTCB's Compounded Sterile Preparation Technician Certification (CSPT), and three years of work experience, will be eligible to earn an Advanced Certified Pharmacy Technician (CPhT-Adv) credential."

Assessment-based certificate programs "evaluate learning outcomes from a PTCB-Recognized Education/Training program, do not expire or require maintenance, and do not award an acronym after the name." There are numerous assessment-based certificate programs, including the Controlled Substances Diversion Prevention Certificate, the Technician Product Verification Certificate (TPV) the Hazardous Drug Management Certificate, and the Medication History Certificate.

Eligibility Requirements for PTCB Certification

There are various requirements for achieving PTCB certification – not just passing the exam. These requirements are:

- You must reside in the United States of America or its territories (U.S.).

- You must comply with all applicable PTCB certification policies (more information at www.ptcbhero.co/policies).

- You must fully disclose all criminal and State Board of Pharmacy registration or licensure actions.

- New (as of 2020): you must complete a PTCB-recognized education/training program OR have equivalent work experience. More on this below.

- And, of course, you must achieve a passing score on the PTCE.

How to participate in a PTCB-recognized education/training program

This requirement was introduced in 2020. You must now complete a PTCB-recognized education/training program OR equivalent work experience in order to be eligible to take the PTCE and then gain your certification once you've passed the exam.

If you wish to go down the "recognized education/training program" route, PTCB has a directory of all recognized programs on its website: www.ptcb-hero.co/directory.

Ideally, you will complete your education/training program before applying to schedule your PTCE. However, you can apply to schedule your exam before you have completed the program, on the condition that you have less than 60 days remaining of your education/training. In this scenario, you will be authorized to schedule and take the PTCE prior to the completion of your program. Be aware that you will not be granted certification until PTCB has received evidence that you've completed your program (which must be within 60 days of your exam date). Acceptable evidence/documentation includes:

- Certificate of completion indicating your name, the education/ training program title, and completion date

- Letter from an education/training provider official on official letterhead, indicating your name, the education/training program title, and completion date

- Unofficial transcript or diploma

For a detailed description of acceptable evidence/documentation, visit www.ptcbhero.co/idproof.

If you wish to complete work experience instead of an approved education/training program...

Instead of completing an approved education/training program, you may prefer to complete equivalent work experience as a pharmacy technician (minimum 500 hours). This alternative path is primarily intended for experienced technicians who are unable to attend a PTCB-recognized program or have already gained much of the required knowledge through work experience.

About the **PTCB Exam**

How to Apply for the PTCE

The PTCE is your final step toward becoming a nationally certified pharmacy technician: once you have passed the exam, you'll have fulfilled all the necessary requirements for PTCB certification. (See the chapter called "Eligibility Requirements" for more.)

If you're a first-time candidate and/or you don't yet have a PTCB account, your first step is to register for a PTCB account:

1. Visit the PTCB Portal at www.ptcbhero.co/portal, then click "Get Started" to register as a new user.
2. On subsequent screens, add all the information required, such as your name, your chosen password for the account, your date of birth, email address, and mailing address. You'll also need to review and agree to the organization's terms and conditions and privacy policy.
3. Once you have reviewed your profile summary, click "Continue." A "PTCB Account Creation Confirmation" page will appear.

Once you've set up your account (or if you already have an account), log into your PTCB account to submit a new application to take the PTCE:

1. Visit www.ptcbhero.co/portal again and enter your username and password.
2. Click the application link under "Earn Your CPhT Certification".
3. Complete the application and application/exam fee payment (which costs $129 as of 2021). Note: the application process involves providing details of your education/training program or work experience. You will be unable to complete the application unless you can provide details of this.
4. When your application has been approved, you'll receive an email with the subject line "Authorization to Schedule." The email will contain instructions on how to schedule and take the PTCE. You can

schedule your appointment online or through Pearson Vue. The exam is administered year-round.

Important: once you receive authorization to schedule your appointment, this authorization lasts for 90 days – meaning you must take your exam within 90 days of receiving the authorization. If the authorization period expires before you take the exam, you will forfeit all fees and must reapply to take the exam. (You do, however, have the option to extend your exam authorization period for an additional 90 days through your PTCB account. You are limited to two 90-day extensions.)

Frequently asked questions about the PTCE application process

Q: Can I apply to take the PTCE before I've completed my education/ training program?

A: Yes – on the condition that you have less than 60 days remaining of your education/training. In this scenario, you will be authorized to schedule and take the PTCE prior to the completion of your program, but you will not be granted certification until PTCB has received evidence that you've completed your program (which must be within 60 days of your exam date).

Acceptable evidence/documentation includes:

- Certificate of completion indicating your name, the education/ training program title, and completion date
- Letter from an education/training provider official on official letterhead, indicating your name, the education/training program title, and completion date
- Unofficial transcript or diploma

For a detailed description of acceptable evidence/documentation, visit www.ptcbhero.co/idproof.

Q: Where are the exams administered/held?

A: PTCB exams are administered at over 1,400 Pearson VUE test centers nationwide, although not all test centres administer specific PTCB exams. To find your nearest one, visit the Pearson VUE website (www.ptcbhero.co/pearson) or call (866) 902-0593. Most test centers are open Monday through Saturday, during normal business hours.

Q: Can I reschedule or cancel my exam appointment?

A: Yes – you can reschedule or cancel your exam appointment for no fee as long as you reschedule at least one business day (24 hours) before the scheduled exam appointment. For example, if your exam is scheduled for 11:00 on a Monday, you must reschedule or cancel by 11:00 the previous Friday. To reschedule, click the "My scheduled exam appointment" link within your PTCB account or call Pearson VUE on (866) 902-0593.

If you do not reschedule or cancel within 24 hours of your scheduled exam appointment (or if you fail to show up for your exam), you will forfeit all fees.

For more information, visit www.ptcbhero.co/reschedule.

Q: What should I do if I cannot attend on the day of my exam due to an emergency? Will I still have to forfeit all fees?

A: If an emergency occurs on the day of your exam (meaning you cannot attend), you can submit an Emergency Withdrawal Request Form along with official documentation of the emergency – ensuring the form is received by PTCB no later than 48 hours after the last day of your 90-day authorization period. Visit www.ptcbhero.co/reschedule for more information, and to download the form.

Q: Once I've passed the exam, will I achieve PTCB certification?

A: Yes, but you'll have to wait a bit! While your unofficial/preliminary result will appear on the screen immediately after you've taken the exam, this isn't official or final. Your official/final exam result will be posted to your PTCB account on the PTCB Portal within three weeks – and, if you've passed, you'll be able to download your PTCB certificate through your PTCB account. View the chapter called "Exam Results, and How to Interpret Them" for more information.

Q: I can't complete my application online; what should I do?

A: According to PTCB, "A paper application is only available to those with a disability or hardship that precludes using the online application. Requests to use the paper application must be submitted in writing to PTCB and include appropriate documentation of the disability or hardship."

Q: I have a criminal record. Am I still allowed to become certified?

A: When you apply to take the PTCE, you must disclose "Yes" if you were, or are currently "the subject of a: charge, complaint, or conviction related to a criminal matter; or, investigation or discipline by a government agency or other authority such as a State Board of Pharmacy, a professional association, or a credentialing organization."

You will then be asked to provide, as part of the application, "a complete detailed explanation of the circumstances related to this response and copies of all final dispositions or resolutions related to these matters." You must further agree that a "failure to include the required explanation and documentation may delay the processing of my Application, or result in the rejection of my Application." (You must submit supporting documentation within 30 days of the application submission date.)

PTCB will then apply specific criteria in order to decide if you are still eligible. For example, the organization will look at "The relationship of the criminal or disciplinary matter to the applicant's professional activities and/or ethical responsibilities," in addition to "The severity of the criminal and disciplinary matter" and "Whether the criminal or disciplinary matter is part of a pattern of criminal, unethical, or otherwise improper conduct." After applying these and other criteria, PTCB will then determine if you are a) eligible for certification, b) temporarily or permanently disqualified from eligibility, and/or c) subject to eligibility conditions.

Q: How do I pay the application fee?

A: The application and exam fee costs $129 as of 2021. You pay online as part of the application process by credit/debit card (American Express, Discover, MasterCard, or VISA).

Q: I have a disability/medical condition, and special provisions will need to be made for me during the exam. What should I do?

A: PTCB complies with the Americans with Disabilities Act of 1990 (ADA) and will "make reasonable testing accommodations for certification candidates when appropriate, and consistent with such legal requirements." If you have a documented disability that limits your sensory, manual, speaking, or other functional skills (including a disability that impairs your ability to arrive at, read, or otherwise complete, the examination), PTCB will provide the necessary testing accommodations (including additional time to complete the exam or the use of approved auxiliary aids).

Note: if you require a testing accommodation (which includes the need to bring your own medical equipment into the testing room), you must do so during the application process by downloading the "Testing Accommodations Form" and submitting it within 30 days of submitting your certification application. The form can be downloaded from this page: www.ptcbhero.co/accommodations.

Format, Content, and Timing
of the Exam

What is the format of the PTCB exam?

The PTCB exam is called the Pharmacy Technician Certification Exam (PTCE). It is a computer-based exam with 90 multiple-choice questions – 80 of which are scored, and 10 of which are unscored. Unscored questions are placed randomly throughout the exam, and you won't know which ones they are. Each multiple-choice question will have four possible answers; you must select which you think is the correct answer for each question.

What are "unscored questions"?

Unscored questions do not have an impact on your final score, so it doesn't matter if you get them right or wrong (only scored questions will be used to calculate your exam score). These are included to assess the quality and relative difficulty of the questions themselves, with the aim of determining whether these questions should be used in future PTCB exams. For example, if most people get a particular unscored question wrong, it implies there's something wrong with it and it should not be included as a scored question on future exams.

How much time will I have for the exam?

You'll have one hour and 50 minutes to answer the questions, although the entire exam is two hours long. This is because you'll be given five minutes at the start to read the tutorial (which contains important instructions on how to navigate the exam questions), and there will be five minutes at the end for a post-exam survey.

Which topics are covered in the exam?

PTCB implemented its most recent update to the exam in 2020, with questions categorized across four knowledge domains. (Note: questions are randomly distributed throughout the exam – i.e. they are not presented in the order of the knowledge domains below.)

The four knowledge domains are:

- Medications (40% of the exam's content)

- Federal Requirements (12.5%)

- Patient Safety and Quality Assurance (26.25%)

- Order Entry and Processing (21.25%)

(For a complete breakdown of the subtopics within each knowledge domain, read the chapter called "How to Structure Your Study Sessions.")

Important: if you see any study guides or practice tests from other companies that mention different numbers or knowledge domains, they are **outdated** and should not be used.

Exam Results and How to Interpret Them

When will I find out the results of my exam?

As soon as you have completed the post-exam survey, your unofficial/ preliminary exam result will appear on the screen. This result is an indication of your performance, but it isn't final – you'll have to wait for the official exam result for that.

Your official/final exam result will be posted to your PTCB account on the PTCB Portal within three weeks (see the chapter called "How to Apply for the PTCE" for more information on the PTCB Portal). Your result will show how well you performed in each knowledge domain, which is helpful for discovering where your strengths and weaknesses lie. If you don't pass, you'll know which areas to focus on before the next exam.

How is the exam scored?

Not everyone who takes the PTCB exam in the same year will receive the same exact set of questions. The exam is designed to test the same content, but the number of "difficult" questions can fluctuate. As a result, the PTCE is scored using a "scaled scoring system," which takes the exam variability into account. Scaled scores are comparable across candidates despite differences in exam difficulty, which allows all candidates to be held to the same scoring standard.

A passing score on the PTCE is 1,400 or higher. The possible score range is 1,000 to 1,600.

What happens if I pass?

If you meet all eligibility requirements (see the "Eligibility Requirements" chapter) and pass your PTCB exam, you can download your certificate through your PTCB account on the PTCB Portal. You can also download a digital badge, which can be displayed in your email signature, resume, and on social media sites. Additionally, you can choose to order a fine paper certificate with a wallet-sized card (for a small fee) from your account.

Remember: to maintain certification, you must renew your certification every two years by completing 20 hours of Continuing Education in a pharmacy-related subject matter. Visit www.ptcbhero.co/renew for more information.

What happens if I fail?

Once you've read and absorbed this book, it's unlikely you'll fail the PTCE! If, however, you find yourself in that position, don't worry: you can apply to retake the exam 60 days after your first attempt. If you don't pass your second attempt, you must wait a further 60 days to apply for your third attempt. After your third attempt, you must wait six months for your fourth attempt. You're not limited to a finite number of exam attempts, but you will have to pay each time you re-apply.

(After four attempts, you'll need to provide PTCB with evidence that you've completed "acceptable preparation activities," which the organization will review and approve before you can apply for additional attempts. Don't worry, though: you'll pass before you reach this stage! For more information on the PTCB's retake policy, visit www.ptcbhero.co/retake.)

Exam Preparation Tips

How to Structure Your Study Sessions

This book contains the KEY facts you need to know and nothing else – ensuring you don't waste any time on unnecessary information. There's no filler, no fluff, and no unnecessary details – allowing you to learn and memorize everything much more quickly than any other book or study guide out there.

But you'll be setting yourself up for failure if your study strategy involves simply skimming this book the night before the exam. Yes: it contains all the need-to-know information, but you *need to know that information*! And you need to understand it too – to enable you to answer questions that are asked in an unfamiliar way, or questions that are structured in a way that's different from what you're used to.

Daunted? Don't be. In this chapter you'll learn how to structure your study sessions to ensure you're prepared and ready to pass on exam day. Let's get started…

1: Start with the official PTCB breakdown of the knowledge domains

Here is a full breakdown of the knowledge domains (repeated from earlier in the book):

1: Medications (40% of PTCE content)

1.1: Generic names, brand names, and classifications of medications

1.2: Therapeutic equivalence

1.3: Common and life-threatening drug interactions and contraindications (e.g., drug-disease, drug-drug, drug-dietary supplement, drug-laboratory, drug-nutrient)

1.4*: Strengths/dose, dosage forms, routes of administration, special handling and administration instructions, and duration of drug therapy

1.5: Common and severe medication side effects, adverse effects, and allergies

1.6: Indications of medications and dietary supplements

1.7*: Drug stability (e.g., oral suspensions, insulin, reconstitutables, injectables, vaccinations)

1.8: Narrow therapeutic index (NTI) medications

1.9: Physical and chemical incompatibilities related to non-sterile compounding and reconstitution

1.10: Proper storage of medications (e.g., temperature ranges, light sensitivity, restricted access)

2: Federal Requirements (12.5% of PTCE content)

2.1: Federal requirements for handling and disposal of non-hazardous, hazardous, and pharmaceutical substances and waste

2.2*: Federal requirements for controlled substance prescriptions (i.e., new, refill, transfer) and DEA controlled substance schedules

2.3: Federal requirements (e.g., DEA, FDA) for controlled substances (i.e., receiving, storing, ordering, labeling, dispensing, reverse distribution, take-back programs, and loss or theft of)

2.4*: Federal requirements for restricted drug programs and related medication processing (e.g., pseudoephedrine, Risk Evaluation and Mitigation Strategies [REMS])

2.5: FDA recall requirements (e.g., medications, devices, supplies, supplements, classifications)

3: Patient Safety and Quality Assurance (26.25% of PTCE content)

3.1: High-alert/risk medications and look-alike/sound-alike [LASA] medications

3.2: Error prevention strategies (e.g., prescription or medication order to correct patient, Tall Man lettering, separating inventory, leading and trailing zeros, bar code usage, limit use of error-prone abbreviations)

3.3*: Issues that require pharmacist intervention (e.g., drug utilization review [DUR], adverse drug event [ADE], OTC recommendation, therapeutic substitution, misuse, adherence, post-immunization follow-up, allergies, drug interactions)

3.4: Event reporting procedures (e.g., medication errors, adverse effects, and product integrity, MedWatch, near miss, root-cause analysis [RCA])

3.5*: Types of prescription errors (e.g., abnormal doses, early refill, incorrect quantity, incorrect patient, incorrect drug)

3.6: Hygiene and cleaning standards (e.g., handwashing, personal protective equipment [PPE], cleaning counting trays, countertop, and equipment)

4: Order Entry and Processing (21.25% of PTCE content)

4.1*: Procedures to compound non-sterile products (e.g., ointments, mixtures, liquids, emulsions, suppositories, enemas)

4.2*: Formulas, calculations, ratios, proportions, alligations, conversions, Sig codes (e.g., b.i.d., t.i.d., Roman numerals), abbreviations, medical terminology, and symbols for days supply, quantity, dose, concentration, dilutions

4.3*: Equipment/supplies required for drug administration (e.g., package size, unit dose, diabetic supplies, spacers, oral and injectable syringes)

4.4*: Lot numbers, expiration dates, and National Drug Code (NDC) numbers

4.5: Procedures for identifying and returning dispensable, non-dispensable, and expired medications and supplies (e.g., credit return, return to stock, reverse distribution)

Some or all of this statement reflects calculation-based knowledge.

Start by paying attention to the weighting of each knowledge domain. As you can see, "Medications" takes up 40% of the exam's content – so be sure to devote a particularly large chunk of time to reminding yourself of the key aspects of the domain.

Next, look at the topics within each domain. How well do you know and understand each of them? You could write a percentage amount next to each topic, representing how well you think you know it. Then, when you go through the rest of the book, devote time to really digging into those topics you're less familiar with. You can update each "topic percentage" as you improve your understanding of it – a nice, visual way of marking your progress.

2: Discover which study method suits you best – and use it

According to experts, different people have different learning styles – meaning some people retain information more easily when it is presented via one format or method, while others prefer a totally different style. While there's some disagreement on precisely how many learning styles there are (anywhere up to seven!), we've found that four learning styles in particular seem to cover most students. These are:

- Visual learning

- Reading/writing learning

- Auditory learning

- Kinesthetic learning

Visual learners enjoy using pictures, images, and graphics for learning. In order to absorb information and "make it stick," visual learners like to rely on drawing, doodling, color-coding, and making posters. They tend to process information better when it is presented as a whole rather than piecemeal – so it's a good idea to use charts and diagrams that summarize information rather than sequential slides of information.

Reading/writing learners enjoy the written word. Whether it's PowerPoint slides, textbooks, or text-heavy websites, they can synthesize the information well. They also tend to absorb information and recall it easily later by writing things down – so they do well when taking copious notes during lectures, for example.

Auditory learners often struggle to read things silently, and may move their lips or talk quietly when writing something down. They learn better through songs, audiobooks, podcasts, stories, and discussion. Another great way for auditory learners to learn is by absorbing the information (e.g. by listening to it or reading it out loud to themselves), then teaching that information to someone else.

Kinesthetic learners benefit from using their bodies to learn. They need to be involved in making projects, role playing, and learning while standing or moving around. If you struggle to sit still and find yourself pacing while trying to absorb new information, there's a good chance you're a kinesthetic learner!

It's unlikely you'll fit neatly into one specific type of learning: you might find you like to combine listening to information then writing it down, for example. Even so, knowing these learning styles and identifying which appeal to you will help you structure your study time better. If you know you're at least partially an auditory learner, you could read out sections of this book and record them, then listen to the recordings later. Or if you know you enjoy learning visually, you can create charts and diagrams out of some of the information.

3: Make sure you're retaining the information

Whichever learning style you prefer, you will need to assess if it's effective – that is, you must make sure that you're actually retaining the information. So how can you check?

Flashcards are a useful first step. You can create your own, or there are plenty to buy online (make sure they reflect the most recent changes to the PTCB exam). Take them everywhere you go, and use any spare moment to review them. If you start to find particular flashcards "easy" (i.e. you know them and understand them right away), remove them from the pack so you have more time to focus on the topics you find trickier.

Next up: practice tests. **This book has an accompanying online study package called PTCB Hero Online (www.ptcbhero.co)**, which contains hundreds of realistic practice questions. With our practice questions, you can focus on one knowledge domain at a time, or mix them all up. You'll also get detailed explanations of the correct answers – so you can learn as you go along.

After you've worked your way through the practice questions and you feel confident about your knowledge, it's time to test your expertise with a simulated exam! **PTCB Hero Online** contains two simulated exams, which replicate the real-life exam you'll be taking. They contain a true representation of the types of questions you'll be asked in the real thing, and they'll be timed – allowing you to get used to the full exam experience. You'll also receive detailed explanations of the correct answers afterward (which won't happen on the real exam).

Buy PTCB Hero Online and get:

- **Hundreds of practice questions** with complete explanations of the correct answers (you can focus on one knowledge domain at a time, or mix them up)

- **Two simulated exam**s with complete explanations of the correct answers

- **A condensed version of this book** – so you can learn on your device whenever you have a spare moment

Visit www.ptcbhero.co and enter 30OFFNOW at checkout for 30% off.

Acceptable Proof of Identity
to Take to the Exam

The most important item to take with you to the exam is proof of identity: a valid, unexpired, government-issued identification (ID) with a photograph and signature. If you do not arrive at the test center with acceptable ID, you will not be allowed to take the exam and you will forfeit all fees.

The following are approved forms of ID:

- Passport/passport card

- Government-issued driver's license or identification card

- Government-issued driving learner's permit

- Military ID

- Permanent resident card (i.e. a Green Card)

- US Department of Homeland Security-issued Employment Authorization Card

The name on your ID must match the name that appears in your PTCB account – although there are some exceptions. For example, you will still be allowed to test if your name contains a hyphen on one document but not the other. Also, names with initials and reversed names are acceptable (J Smith and John Smith/Smith J. and J. Smith/etc). For a full list of exceptions, visit www.ptcbhero.co/exceptions.

If your ID does not contain a signature, you must present a valid, unexpired secondary form of ID that contains your first and last name and includes your signature. Examples of secondary ID include:

- Social security card

- Credit card
- ATM/debit card
- Employee/school ID

Items Allowed (and Not Allowed) in the Exam Room

PTCB has strict rules around what can be taken and not taken into the exam room. If you need a particular item that isn't on the "allowed" list (such as specific medical equipment or breast-pumping equipment), you must make a request during the application process by downloading the "Request for Testing Accommodations Form" and submitting it within 30 days of submitting your certification application. The form can be downloaded from this page: www.ptcbhero.co/accommodations.

Items allowed in the exam room

These items are "comfort aids" and do not require pre-approval. They will be allowed in the exam room after a visual inspection by exam center staff.

Medicine and medical devices

- Auto-injectors – e.g. EpiPen

- Bandages

- Braces (neck, back, wrist, leg, or ankle braces)

- Casts – including slings for broken/sprained arms and other injury-related items that cannot be removed

- Cough drops (must be unwrapped and not in a bottle/container)

- Eye drops

- Eye patches

- Eyeglasses (without the case)

- Glucose tablets (does not include hard candy) – must be unwrapped and not in a bottle/container

- Handheld (non-electronic) magnifying glass (without the case)

- Hearing aids/cochlear implant (if the aids/implant includes an accompanying remote-control device, this may not be taken into the exam room; if you wish to take the device into the room, you will need to gain approval via the Request for Testing Accommodations Form mentioned above)

- Inhaler

- Medical alert bracelet (note: if your medical alert bracelet has a USB port, you must not plug it into the computer workstation)

- A medical device that is attached to your body or not easily removable, such as an insulin pump or a continuous glucose monitor (note: the device must be inaudible, and – if it includes a remote-control device – this must not be taken into the exam room unless permission has been granted via the Testing Accommodation Form in advance)

- TENS unit

- Spinal cord stimulator

- Face mask and/or gloves

- Medical foot stool – for the purpose of supporting an injured leg/foot (the stool must be non-skid, have a metal base, and can be no larger than 14 x 14 x 12)

- Nasal drops/spray

- Oxygen tank

- Pillow/cushion

- Pills such as Tylenol and aspirin (must be unwrapped and not in a bottle/container)

- Pills that MUST remain in their packaging (e.g. to prevent loss of potency); you should expect staff at the center to examine such medications thoroughly.

Mobility devices

- Canes

- Crutches

- Motorized scooters/chairs

- Walkers

- Wheelchairs

Other approved items

- Tissues/Kleenex (note: these will be provided by the testing center – you must not bring your own)

- Earplugs and noise-reducing/canceling headphones

Items not allowed in the exam room

- Electronic gadgets including cell phones, PDAs, calculators, and translators

- Outer clothing such as jackets

- Hats

- Barrettes, clips that are bigger than a quarter inch, and hair bands wider than a half inch

- Personal calculators (a calculator is built into the PTCB exam, and you may also request to use a hand-held calculator from the test center)

During the Exam: Some Tips

Learning, understanding, and remembering all the information required for passing the exam is your crucial first step in passing the exam. (The "Knowledge Domains" part of this book contains ALL the information you need to know for the exam.) But knowing and understanding the content is only part of it. You also need to have the right set of exam-taking skills – to make sure you don't get stuck on terminology, panicked about timing, or stumped by question phrasing.

This chapter gives you tips on improving your exam-taking skills, so that you can maximize your chances of answering each question correctly.

1: Read carefully

Don't skim! Read through each question carefully to ensure you've fully understood what's being asked. For example, read the following question:

Q: Which of the following methods can contribute to a reduction of medication errors?

A: Omit the leading zero

B: Use a trailing zero

C: Write "daily" in the sig

D: Write IU for International Unit

Many people misread this question as "Which of the following methods can contribute to medication errors?" – and as a result, they select an incorrect option from the list of possible answers. (The correct answer is "C.")

Here's another example of a question that's frequently answered incorrectly:

Q: Which of the following medications must be refrigerated prior to reconstitution and administration?

A: Epoetin alfa

B: Vancomycin

C: Azithromycin

D: Ceftriaxone

You must keep in mind that the question asks for the refrigeration requirement **prior to reconstitution and administration.** Vancomycin, azithromycin, and ceftriaxone vials can be stored at room temperature, but once they are reconstituted and mixed with a base solution such as normal saline, the final products must be refrigerated. The only medication that requires refrigeration **prior** to reconstitution is epoetin alfa.

2: Remember that there's often more than one "reasonable" answer to a question

The PTCB exam isn't intended to catch you out or trick you, but each question will contain four possible answers – and the exam writers will often include *at least* two reasonable answer choices for each question. If you find yourself zeroing in on one answer as THE definite response, be careful: your first assumption may be incorrect. Take your time and look at all the possible answers – don't just pick the first one that looks right without reading the others.

Here's an example question that has two reasonable answers:

_____ must be taken 30 to 60 minutes before a meal, usually once a day.

a)   Pantoprazole

b) Hydrochlorothiazide

c) Sucralfate

d) Lisinopril

Correct answer: a) Pantoprazole

Explanation:

If you're not careful in reading all of the answer choices, you might select "sucralfate." Sucralfate should be given an hour before a meal, but it's usually dosed 3 to 4 times per day. So, the correct answer to this question is pantoprazole. Pantoprazole is a proton pump inhibitor (PPI) which provides optimal effects when administered 30 to 60 minutes before a meal and is usually dosed once a day.

3: Try to predict the answer

This tip doesn't work for all questions, but it's particularly useful when answering math-based questions. When you read a math-based question, stop before you reach the answer choices and try to predict or work out what the answer will be. That way, you'll feel more certain of your answer choice – and it's less likely you'll be distracted by other possible answers because you'll know exactly which answer you're looking for.

4: Eliminate all incorrect answers until you're left with the right one

This tip is handy for all questions, but particularly those where you're not sure of the answer. Rather than trying to find the correct answer choice, turn things around: seek out all the choices that definitely don't answer the question.

If you're unable to eliminate all answer choices, move on and return to this question later (see tip below). You may find you're still unable to eliminate all answer choices, but let's say you're left with two: you now have far better odds of getting it correct (50%) than if you were to randomly select from four (where your odds are 25%).

5: Remember that an answer choice might be factually true but incorrect

You want to select the choice that answers the question – not the one that happens to be factually true.

Here's an example question to clarify this tip:

What is the smallest volume of liquid that can be measured in a 50-mL graduated cylinder?

a)   3 mL

b)   5 mL

c)   10 mL

d)   20 mL

Correct answer: c) 10 mL

Explanation:

Without any knowledge on this subject, it could be reasoned that "3 mL" is, in fact, the smallest volume listed in the answer choices. But as a pharmacy technician, you should know that you wouldn't be able to accurately measure out 3 mL using a 50-mL graduated cylinder. The amount of liquid to be measured in a graduated cylinder shouldn't be less than 20% of its total capacity. We arrive at the correct answer by calculating that 20% of 50 mL = 10 mL.

6: If you're stuck, move on

Don't spend tons of time on questions that stump you: you may end up running out of time before you reach questions you *can* answer.

A far better approach is to work your way through the exam, answering questions you know. Then return to any you were stuck on. This strategy helps in three ways: 1) you'll have answered all the questions you *can* answer, giving you a better chance of a passing grade; 2) you'll feel more calm and relaxed, which means you'll be a in a better frame of mind to attack questions you find trickier; 3) reading through all the other questions may help to jog your memory about topics you struggled with the first time around.

7: Pace yourself

It's easy to feel daunted and overwhelmed when you first start the exam: 90 questions all needing to be read, contemplated, and answered. But don't rush: you have plenty of time. If you find you have less time than you think toward the end of the exam, stay calm: it's far better that you use those minutes to answer a few questions correctly than to rush through and answer everything incorrectly.

8: Check your work

Once you've answered all the questions, there should be enough time to go back through the entire exam and double check your answer selections. Even though you've read each question carefully, eliminated incorrect answers, and made use of all the other tips on this list, there's still a chance you made a careless mistake.

9: Get into the zone

You might be in a room with other candidates, and those candidates may have a habit of tapping their foot, blowing their nose, or doing all manner of other distracting things! To help you focus, consider taking some noise-canceling headphones or earplugs with you.

10: Make sure you've had enough sleep the night before!

According to multiple scientific studies, pulling an all-nighter of study is extremely counterproductive! For example, a University of Minnesota study discovered a "significant positive correlation between amount of sleep per night with GPA, and a significant negative correlation between average number of days per week that students obtained less than five hours of sleep and GPA" (www.ptcbhero.co/minnesota). And according to research reported by Science Daily, all-nighters rely on short-term memory – which means the information you absorb can disappear before the exam (www.ptcbhero.co/sciencedaily).

Your brain isn't designed to absorb vast amounts of information on no sleep and then retain it for the exam. Your brain also isn't designed to perform well late at night.

The best way to prepare for your exam? Study in short bursts, several times a day, for several days before the exam. Read the chapter called "How to Structure Your Study Sessions" for more tips on how to prepare.

Introduction to the
Four Knowledge Domains

So What's Changed?

The content outline of the PTCE was revised and updated in January 2020 – and the changes are significant. This means that if you've been looking at study materials written or published prior to 2020, stop! Those materials are outdated and should not be used. (In fact, even if the study material says that it's relevant for "2020–2021," double check that it's not based on the old content outline.)

The new content outline contains four knowledge domains (instead of the previous nine), in order to focus on core, essential knowledge that applies across practice settings. This new content structure ensures that the PTCE is more relevant as an entry-level credential for various medical establishments, making it a more useful certification for newly qualified Certified Pharmacy Technicians (CPhTs) and employers alike.

The rest of this book focuses on those four knowledge domains that you'll need to know in detail for your exam. They are:

- Medications (40% of the exam's content)

- Federal Requirements (12.5%)

- Patient Safety and Quality Assurance (26.25%)

- Order Entry and Processing (21.25%)

For each domain, we've included the KEY facts and nothing else – because we don't want you wasting any time on unnecessary information. Your job is to learn the knowledge domains in the way that suits you best (see the chapter on "How to Structure Your Study Sessions"). To *really* cement your learning, you can choose to test yourself with practice tests and simulated exams from **PTCB Hero Online**.

Remember: **PTCB Hero Online** contains hundreds of practice questions PLUS two simulated exams (which replicate the real-life exams you'll be taking). All the practice questions and simulated exam questions include detailed explanations of the correct answers afterward. Visit **www.ptcbhero.co** and enter 30OFFNOW at checkout for 30% off.

Now… it's time to get started with those knowledge domains! Let's go!

Knowledge Domain 1:

Medications

Pharmacology

Pharmacology is the study of drugs and their effects on living organisms. Clinical pharmacology is the study of how drugs work in the human body. Studying pharmacology requires a basic understanding of anatomy, physiology, chemistry, and pathology.

There are two major branches of pharmacology: pharmacodynamics (what the drug does to the body) and pharmacokinetics (what the body does to the drug).

Pharmacokinetics (PK)

Pharmacokinetics (PK) is a branch of pharmacology that studies what the body does to a drug. How a drug moves into, through, and out of the body is described by studying its PK.

There are four important components of PK: absorption, distribution, metabolism, and excretion. (Use the acronym "ADME" to remember.)

1. Absorption: the process of drugs entering the body into the bloodstream.
2. Distribution: the process where the drug is distributed or dispersed throughout the body.
3. Metabolism: the process where the drug is broken down by the body, usually in the liver or gastrointestinal (GI) tract. This results in metabolites, which can be inactive or active.
4. Excretion: after metabolism, the drug is eliminated from the body.

Bioavailability

Bioavailability is an important concept of PK. It is defined as the amount of the administered drug that reaches the blood circulation and can be used by the body. For example, a drug that is administered intravenously (into a vein) has a bioavailability of 100%. But drugs that are administered orally (by mouth) must pass through the digestive tract and have a reduced bioavailability. That is, a reduced percentage of the dose actually reaches the bloodstream.

When two drugs have the same bioavailability, they are deemed to be bioequivalent (BE) – i.e. these drugs are absorbed equally into the body.

Approved drug products are considered to be therapeutic equivalents if they have demonstrated BE and can be expected to have the same clinical effect and safety profile. The FDA maintains a publication of approved drug products and their therapeutic equivalents known as the Orange Book.

Route of administration

Route of administration is one of the main factors that affects a drug's bioavailability. The most frequently used routes of administration include:

Description	Administration route	Abbreviation (if any)
By mouth	Oral	PO
Under the tongue	Sublingual	SL
Between the gums & cheek	Buccal	N/A

Into the muscle	Intramuscular	IM
Under the skin	Subcutaneous	SC
Into the vein	Intravenous	IV
Into the spinal cord spaces	Intrathecal	N/A
Into the rectum	Rectal	PR
Into the vagina	Vaginal	PV
Through the skin	Transdermal	N/A
On the skin	Topical	N/A
Into the nostril	Intranasal	N/A
Into the lungs	Inhalation	N/A
Into the ear	Otic	AS (left ear), AD (right), AU (both)
Into the eye	Ocular or ophthalmic	OS (left eye), OD (right), OU (both)

A note about abbreviations: Some institutions and organizations recommend against the use of medical abbreviations. The concern is that medical abbreviations could be misinterpreted and lead to medical errors. In practice, be sure to follow your institution's guidelines.

Pharmacodynamics (PD) is the opposite of PK: it is the study of the biochemical and physiological effects of drugs on the body. PD is important because it helps us learn what the optimum dose of a drug should be – one that limits side effects while maximizing the clinical effect of the drug.

Pharmacodynamics (PD)

Receptors

For drugs to affect the body, they have to reach their target cells or tissues. They do this by interacting with receptors, which are proteins located inside the cells or on the cell surface.

Agonist and antagonist drug molecules

Most drugs fit into two general categories that describe how they interact with receptors at the molecular level: agonists and antagonists.

Agonist drug molecules

Agonist drug molecules mimic normal physiological processes in the body. When an agonist drug molecule binds to a receptor, it activates the receptor and generates a response.

Imagine a drug as a key and a receptor as the lock. The key fits inside the lock and turns it to open the door (i.e. it activates the receptor). This mechanism is known as agonism.

For example, albuterol is a beta-2 agonist. Albuterol and other beta-2 agonists are indicated to treat asthma and other pulmonary diseases. Albuterol is the key and the beta-2 receptor in the lungs is the lock. When albuterol binds to and activates beta-2 receptors, bronchodilation takes place, relieving symptoms such as shortness of breath.

Antagonist drug molecules

Antagonist drug molecules are designed to inhibit or block an agonist from activating a receptor. Imagine the antagonist as a key that fits into the lock but doesn't have the right shape to unlock it. When the wrong key is occupying this space, it prevents the proper key (the agonist) from getting into the same lock. These actions of the agonist are blocked by the presence of the antagonist in the receptor.

For example, if a patient has taken a life-threatening overdose of an opioid, such as morphine, they can be prescribed naloxone, an opioid receptor antagonist. Naloxone quickly blocks all the opioid receptors in the body, thus preventing morphine from binding to them. If administered promptly, naloxone can prevent death from an opioid overdose.

Neurotransmitters

Neurotransmitters are brain chemicals that send messages to the body by binding with specific receptors. Some examples of neurotransmitters are dopamine, epinephrine, histamine, and serotonin. Agonist drugs often mimic neurotransmitters, and antagonist drugs often inhibit them.

Therapeutic index (TI)

The therapeutic index (TI) of a drug indicates the range of doses at which a medication is both effective and safe. Drugs with a narrow therapeutic index (NTI) have a very small window between their effective doses and those at which they produce unacceptable adverse effects.

The FDA recommends tight therapeutic drug monitoring of NTI drugs to ensure patient safety and drug efficacy. Therapeutic drug monitoring is done by measuring "trough and peak" drug levels in the patient's blood. Trough is the lowest blood concentration of the drug, while peak is the highest blood concentration of the drug. Trough is drawn before the administration of the next dose, while peak is collected one to several hours after the drug administration, depending on the drug.

Some examples of common NTI drugs are:

- Cyclosporine: immunosuppressant used in organ transplant

- Digoxin: atrial fibrillation drug

- Digitoxin: antiarrhythmic drug

- Fosphenytoin: antiepileptic drug

- Levothyroxine: hypothyroidism drug

- Lithium: bipolar disorder drug

- Phenytoin: antiepileptic drug

- Theophylline: asthma and COPD (chronic obstructive pulmonary disease) drug

- Warfarin: blood thinner

Interactions

Drug interactions involve combinations of a medication with other substances that alter the effects on the body. This can cause unexpected side effects or cause the medication to be more or less potent than intended.

Not all drug interactions are detrimental, but some can be life-threatening.

Definitions to know:

> **Indication**: a reason to use a certain treatment. For example, fluconazole (Diflucan®) is indicated to treat a yeast infection.

> **Contraindication** (opposite of indication): a reason not to use a certain treatment due to the harm that it could cause the patient. For example, sildenafil (Viagra®) is contraindicated in men taking nitrates due to the risk of potentially fatal hypotension.

There are several types of drug interactions: drug-drug interactions, drug-disease interactions, drug-nutrient interactions, drug-herbal interactions, drug-alcohol interactions, and drug-laboratory interactions.

Drug-drug interactions

Drug-drug interactions occur when two or more drugs react with each other. There are four main types:

Addition: the combined effect of two drugs is equal to the sum of the effects of each drug taken alone. In other words, one drug can add to the effects or side effects of another drug.

> Example 1: potassium chloride is a potassium supplement that is indicated to increase potassium, while spironolactone is a potassium-sparing diuretic. Each drug can raise potassium levels when administered alone. But co-administration of these two medications can raise potassium to a harmful level, which can affect heart rhythm.

> Example 2: Selective serotonin reuptake inhibitors (SSRIs) are used to treat depression, and triptans are indicated to treat migraines. Both types of drugs affect serotonin levels. Co-administration of agents from these two drug classes can cause too much serotonin in the blood. This is known as serotonin syndrome, which can be serious and requires immediate medical care.

Antagonism: the action of one drug antagonizes (blocks or works against) the action of another drug.

> For example, naloxone blocks the effects of morphine, as previously described in the explanation of antagonist drugs earlier.

Potentiation: one drug enhances or prolongs the effects of another drug.

> For example, nitrates (such as nitroglycerin) and phosphodiesterase-5 inhibitors (such as sildenafil) both cause increased blood flow (vasodilation). Co-administration of nitroglycerin and sildenafil can cause extreme vasodilation, leading to severe hypotension.

Synergism: the combined effect of two drugs is greater than the sum of the effect of two drugs. That is: "2 + 2 = 5."

> For example, gentamicin and ampicillin have a synergistic interaction. Both gentamicin and ampicillin are antimicrobial agents, but they have different mechanisms of action. They attack different components of the bacteria, leading to superior destruction of the bacteria when co-administered.

Drug-disease interactions

Drug-disease interactions occur when a drug that is intended for therapeutic use causes certain harmful effects because of a disease or pre-existing condition that the patient has. This is because certain diseases or conditions may alter the absorption or elimination of some medications.

Examples include the following:

- Pseudoephedrine is the active ingredient in some over-the-counter (OTC) nasal decongestants due to its vasoconstrictive effect. But this vasoconstrictive effect can also cause peripheral blood vessels to be constricted. This can raise blood pressure and prove dangerous for people with hypertension.

- Laxatives can cause dehydration and electrolyte imbalance, which can lead to acute kidney injury or worsen the symptoms of pre-existing kidney disease.

Drug-nutrient interactions

Drug-nutrient interactions occur when certain foods or beverages increase or decrease the effects of drugs in the body.

For example…

Grapefruit juice is an inhibitor of an enzyme called CYP3A4, which is responsible for the metabolism of many types of medication (including alprazolam, amiodarone, atorvastatin, calcium channel blockers, and carbamazepine). Co-administration of grapefruit juice and these medications will decrease the metabolism of the drugs, leading to an excess amount of drug in the bloodstream and potentially leading to adverse effects.

> For example, when co-administered with atorvastatin, grapefruit juice inhibits CYP3A4, which is the enzyme responsible for breaking down atorvastatin. This could lead to increased adverse effects of atorvastatin such as severe muscle weakness and pain, and signs of liver injury, such as fatigue, jaundice, and dark urine.

Warfarin is a blood thinner, which works by indirectly inhibiting vitamin K (an essential vitamin for blood clotting). Green leafy vegetables are rich in vitamin K, so co-administration of warfarin and green leafy vegetables can reduce the blood-thinning effect of warfarin.

Dairy foods like milk and yogurt contain calcium. Calcium and other minerals such as magnesium, aluminum, and iron can interact with certain medications by binding to them and preventing their absorption. To avoid this interaction, these drugs should be separated from dairy or mineral-containing products (e.g. multi-vitamins, antacids) by at least two to four hours.

Some examples of drugs that interact with calcium and other minerals include:

- Bisphosphonates: alendronate

- Fluoroquinolone antibiotics: ciprofloxacin, levofloxacin

- Levothyroxine

Drug-herbal interactions

Drug-herbal interactions occur when herbal or dietary supplements increase or decrease a drug's effects. It is important to know that "natural" or "plant-based" products are not always safe, especially when co-administered with certain medications.

- Ginkgo biloba, a herbal supplement, increases the risk of bleeding. This could create an additive risk of bleeding when it is co-administered with non-steroidal anti-inflammatory drugs (NSAIDs), warfarin, or clopidogrel (antiplatelet medication).

- St. John's Wort, a herbal supplement used to treat depression, increases the adverse effects of several classes of antidepressants – including SSRIs and serotonin-norepinephrine reuptake inhibitors (SNRIs).

- St. John's Wort also can decrease the effectiveness of HIV antiviral medications.

Drug-alcohol interactions

Drug-alcohol interactions occur for two main reasons: alcohol can have chemical reactions with the drug molecule itself, and/or alcohol can have additive harmful side effects with some drugs that are central nervous system (CNS) depressants. Some examples include:

- Metronidazole (Flagyl®), an antibiotic, is contraindicated with alcohol because of a "disulfiram-like" reaction that causes severe vomiting and stomach pain.

- Opioid analgesics (e.g. oxycodone, tramadol) are contraindicated with alcohol because of the risk of additive CNS depression that could result in excessive sedation, respiratory depression, coma, or death.

Drug-laboratory interactions

Many medications can interfere with laboratory testing and cause incorrect results. It is important for patients to tell their healthcare provider all the medications that they're taking, including prescription medications, over-the-counter (OTC) medicines, and dietary supplements. Without this information, inaccurate or misinterpreted lab test results can lead to missed or wrong diagnoses and unnecessary testing.

Examples include the following:

- Thiazide diuretics and loop diuretics can elevate HDL cholesterol levels.

- Barbiturates, thiazide diuretics, corticosteroids, and oral contraceptives can elevate blood glucose levels.

- Beta-blockers, aspirin, and trimethoprim / sulfamethoxazole can decrease blood sugar.

- Thiazide diuretics, angiotensin-converting-enzyme inhibitors (ACE inhibitors, or ACEIs), NSAIDs, and caffeine can cause hypokalemia (low serum potassium).

Drug Names

How drugs are named

A medication has up to three names: a chemical name, a brand (proprietary) name, and a generic (non-proprietary) name. A chemical name refers to the chemical structure of the drug molecule. Drugs are most often referred to by their brand or generic names.

Brand name

A brand or trade name is assigned to a drug by the manufacturer who developed the drug. The drug is patent-protected for approximately 20 years from the date of the patent application.

For example, Lovenox®, a blood thinner by Sanofi-Aventis U.S. LLC, was first approved by the FDA in 1993. Its generic version, enoxaparin, was approved by the FDA in 2010.

Generic name

After the patent of a brand name drug expires, other drug manufacturers are allowed to produce a generic version – often at a lower price. These generic versions are usually named to identify the drug's active ingredient. A drug's active ingredient is the part of the drug that produces its intended pharmaco-logic effect.

A generic drug is essentially a copy of the active ingredient of a brand-name drug. A generic drug is considered bioequivalent (BE) to its brand name version because it has the same pharmacological effect. The only difference might be the inactive ingredients that do not affect a drug's therapeutic action. Different inactive ingredients may lead to differences in appearance, shape, color, flavor, or release mechanism. These inactive ingredients, also known as excipients, do not contribute to pharmacologic effects.

It is important to know the brand and generic names of frequently pre-scribed medications. Some examples of commonly prescribed brand and generic drug names include:

Brand name	Generic name
Amoxil®	Amoxicillin
Glucophage®	Metformin
Lexapro®	Escitalopram
Lipitor®	Atorvastatin
Percocet®	Oxycodone / acetaminophen
Prinivil®, Zestril®	Lisinopril
Synthroid®	Levothyroxine
Toprol XL®	Metoprolol succinate extended-release
Xanax®	Alprazolam
Zithromax®	Azithromycin

Prefixes, suffixes, and root words

Pharmacy technicians must have a basic knowledge of medical terminology. Medical and pharmacological terms are "built" from smaller components. All medical terms contain a "root," and they might have a prefix, a suffix, or both.

- A prefix is placed at the start of a word to specify its meaning.

- The root is the central part of a word. Some medical terms have more than one root, such as "gastroenteritis."

- A suffix is placed at the end of a word to modify its meaning.

"Pericarditis" is an example of a medical term that contains all three components:

- "peri-" is the prefix, and it means "surrounding."

- "card" is the root, and it means "heart."

- "-itis" is the suffix, and it means "inflammation."

Putting it together, it means "inflammation surrounding the heart."

Common root words

- Card/io: heart

- Carcin/o: cancer

- Cyto: cell

- Enter/o: intestine

- Derma: skin

- Gastr/o: stomach

- Pharyng/o: throat (pharynx)

Common prefixes

- Ab- : away from

- Ad- : toward

- Bi- : both or two

- Epi- : upon

- Macro- : large

- Micro- : small

- Pre- : before

- Post- : after

Common suffixes

- -itis: inflammation

- -lysis: breakdown

- -partum: birth

- -pathy: disease

- -otomy: to cut into

- -scopy: visual examination

Classifications of Medications

A drug class is a term used to describe a group of medications that work in a similar way or have a similar effect. Medications can be classified by their pharmacologic effect, such as "bronchodilators." They can be further classified by their mechanism of action, such as "beta-2 agonists."

This chapter reviews each drug class – and their therapeutic effects and adverse effects on each body system. Commonly used drugs from each class will be listed by their generic and brand names, as well as if there's a suffix that identifies the drug class.

1: Cardiovascular system medications

Angiotensin-converting-enzyme inhibitors (ACE inhibitors or ACEIs)

- Indications: hypertension, congestive heart failure, post-myocardial infarction (heart attack) (due to their cardiac-remodeling characteristics)

- Adverse drug reactions: dry and unproductive cough, angioedema (swelling of face, throat, and tongue), hypotension

- Commonly used ACE inhibitors (-pril suffix):

    - Benazepril (Lotensin®)

    - Captopril (Capoten®)

    - Enalapril (Vasotec®)

- Lisinopril (Prinivil®, Zestril®)ss

- Quinapril (Accupril®)

- Ramipril (Altace®)

Angiotensin II receptor blockers (ARBs)

- Indications: same as ACE inhibitors – hypertension, congestive heart failure, post-myocardial infarction (heart attack) (due to their cardiac-remodeling characteristics)

- Adverse drug reactions: dry cough (significantly less so than ACE inhibitors), angioedema, fatigue

- Commonly used ARBs (-sartan suffix):

  - Candesartan (Atacand®)

  - Irbesartan (Avapro®)

- Losartan (Cozaar®)

- Olmesartan (Benicar®)

- Telmisartan (Micardis®)

- Valsartan (Diovan®)

Antiarrhythmic agents

- Indication: abnormal heart rhythm due to atrial and ventricular fibrillation

- Adverse drug reactions (ADRs): QT prolongation, dizziness, drowsiness

- Commonly used antiarrhythmic agents:

  - Amiodarone (Cordarone®, Pacerone®)

  - Flecainide (Tambacor®)

- Lidocaine (Xylocaine®)

- Quinidine (Quinalan®)

- Propafenone (Rythmol®)

Note: other cardiovascular system medications can also be used as antiarrhythmic agents, including beta-blockers and calcium channel blockers.

Anticoagulants

- Indications: commonly known as blood thinners, they prevent the formation of blood clots (such as deep vein thrombosis (DVT)) and reduce the risk of recurrent stroke

- Adverse drug reactions: bleeding, bruising, fatigue

- Commonly used anticoagulants:

  - Apixaban (Eliquis®)

  - Dabigatran (Pradaxa®)

  - Heparin

  - Rivaroxaban (Xarelto®)

  - Warfarin (Janotoven®, Coumadin® – discontinued in 2020)

Note: the antidote to reverse the effects of warfarin is vitamin K (phytonadione).

Antiplatelet agents

- Indication: prevents platelets from sticking together, which reduces the risk of recurrent myocardial infarction, stroke, or angina

- Adverse drug reactions: bleeding, bruising, stomach irritation

- Commonly used antiplatelet agents:

- Aspirin

- Clopidogrel (Plavix®)

- Prasugrel (Effient®)

- Ticagrelor (Brilinta®)

Beta-blockers (BBs)

- Indications: hypertension, angina (chest pain), myocardial infarction, arrhythmias

- Adverse drug reactions: fatigue, bradycardia (slow heart rate), bronchoconstriction, depression

- Commonly used BBs (-o/lol suffix):

  - Atenolol (Tenormin®)

  - Bisoprolol (Zebeta®)

  - Metoprolol succinate extended-release (Toprol XL®, Kapspargo®)

  - Metoprolol tartrate (Lopressor®)

  - Carvedilol (Coreg®)

  - Propranolol (Inderal®)

Calcium channel blockers (CCBs)

- Indications: hypertension, angina, arrhythmias

- Adverse drug reactions: peripheral edema, palpitations, drowsiness, headache

- Commonly used CCBs (-dipine suffix for most CCBs):

  - Amlodipine (Norvasc®)

  - Felodipine (Plendil®)

- Nifedipine (Procardia®)

- Diltiazem (Dilacor XR®, Cardizem®)

- Verapamil (Calan®, Verelan®)

Cardiac glycosides

- Indications: congestive heart failure, arrhythmias

- Adverse drug reactions: diarrhea, headache, dizziness, vision changes

- Commonly used cardiac glycosides:

  - Digoxin (Lanoxin®)

Cholesterol-lowering drugs

- Indications: hypercholesterolemia, hypertriglyceridemia, reduce risk of recurrent myocardial infarction or stroke, reduce recurrent angina

- Adverse drug reactions: can vary with each subtype but generally include muscle pain or numbness, upset stomach, headache, dizziness

- Commonly used cholesterol-lowering drugs (several subtypes):

  - Bile acid sequestrants:

    - Cholestyramine (Questran®)

    - Colesevelam (Welchol®)

    - Colestipol (Colestid®)

  - Fibric acids:

    - Fenofibrate (Tricor®)

    - Gemfibrozil (Lopid®)

  - HMG-CoA reductase inhibitors (-statin suffix):

    - Atorvastatin (Lipitor®)

- Lovastatin (Mevacor®)

- Pravastatin (Pravachol®)

- Rosuvastatin (Crestor®)

- Simvastatin (Zocor®)

- Omega-3 fatty acids:

  - Icosapent ethyl (Vascepa®)

  - Omega-3-acid ethyl esters (Lovaza®)

- Proprotein convertase subtilisin kexin type 9 (PCSK9) inhibitors:

  - Alirocumab (Praluent®)

  - Evolocumab (Repatha®)

- Other miscellaneous types of cholesterol-lowering agents:

  - Bempedoic acid (Nexletol®)

  - Ezetimibe (Zetia®)

  - Niacin (Niaspan®)

Diuretics

- Indication: enhance diuresis (increased urine production) to alleviate edema-related hypertension

- Adverse drug reactions: orthostatic hypotension, hypokalemia (depending on the type of diuretic)

- Commonly used diuretics:

  - Bumetanide (Bumex®)

  - Furosemide (Lasix®)

  - Hydrochlorothiazide (Hydrodiuril®)

- Spironolactone (Aldactone®)

- Triamterene-hydrochlorothiazide (Dyazide®)

Vasodilators

- Indications: angina, hypertension, congestive heart failure

- Adverse drug reactions: orthostatic hypotension, bradycardia, flushing

- Commonly used vasodilators:

  - Isosorbide dinitrate (Dinitrate SR®)

  - Isosorbide mononitrate (Imdur®)

  - Hydralazine (Apresoline®)

  - Nitroprusside (Nitropress®)

  - Nitroglycerin (Nitrostat®)

2: Digestive system medications

Antacids

- Indications: gastroesophageal reflux disease (GERD), peptic ulcer disease (PUD), occasional indigestion

- Adverse drug reactions: constipation, diarrhea

- Commonly used antacids:

  - Aluminum hydroxide/magnesium hydroxide (Maalox®)

  - Calcium carbonate (Tums®)

  - Magnesium hydroxide (Milk of Magnesia®)

Anti-diarrheal agents

- Indication: diarrhea

- Adverse drug reaction: constipation

- Commonly used anti-diarrheal agents:

  - Bismuth subsalicylate (Pepto Bismol®)

  - Diphenoxylate/atropine (Lomotil®)

  - Loperamide (Imodium®)

Anti-gas agents

- Indications: flatulence, gas pain

- Adverse drug reactions: nausea, vomiting, diarrhea

- Commonly used anti-gas agents:

  - Activated charcoal (CharcoCaps®)

  - Simethicone (Gas-X®)

Anti-inflammatory drugs for gastrointestinal (GI) tract (5-aminosalicylates)

- Indications: ulcerative colitis, Crohn's disease

- Adverse drug reactions: muscle or joint pain / stiffness, nausea, vomiting

- Commonly used anti-inflammatory drugs for GI system (-sala- root):

  - Balsalazide (Colazal®)

  - Mesalamine (Apriso®, Canasa®, others)

  - Sulfasalazine (Azulfidine®)

Anti-nausea agents

- Indications: nausea, vomiting, motion sickness

- Adverse drug reactions: drowsiness, diarrhea

- Commonly used anti-nausea agents:

    - Aprepitant (Emend®)

    - Hydroxyzine (Atarax®)

    - Meclizine (Antivert®)

    - Metoclopramide (Reglan®)

    - Ondansetron (Zofran®)

    - Prochlorperazine (Compazine®)

    - Promethazine (Phenergan®)

    - Scopolamine (Transderm Scop®)

Digestive enzymes

- Indication: digestive intolerances due to digestive enzyme insufficiencies

- Adverse drug reactions: hyperglycemia or hypoglycemia, abdominal pain

- Commonly used digestive enzymes (-ase suffix):

    - Lactase (Lactaid®) – lactose digestive enzyme

    - Pancrelipase (Creon®) – pancreatic digestive enzyme

H_2 receptor antagonists

- Indications: GERD, PUD

- Adverse drug reactions: constipation, dizziness

- Commonly used H2 receptor antagonists (-idine suffix):

    - Cimetidine (Tagamet HB®)

    - Ranitidine (Zantac®) (note: ranitidine was removed from the market by the FDA in April 2020, but it may still appear on your exam)

    - Famotidine (Pepcid®)

Laxative agents

- Indication: constipation
- Adverse drug reactions: nausea, vomiting, diarrhea
- Commonly used laxative agents:

    - Bisacodyl (Dulcolax®)

    - Docusate sodium (Colace®)

    - Lactulose (Enulose®)

    - Polyethylene glycol (Miralax®)

    - Psyllium (Metamucil®)

    - Sennosides (Senokot®)

Mucosal protectants

- Indications: PUD caused by NSAIDs (misoprostol), maintenance therapy for duodenal ulcers (sucralfate)
- Adverse drug reaction: headache
- Commonly used mucosal protectants:

    - Misoprostol (Cytotec®)

    - Sucralfate (Carafate®)

Proton pump inhibitors (PPIs)

- Indications: GERD, erosive esophagitis, as an adjunct treatment of H. pylori

- Adverse drug reactions: abdominal pain, constipation, diarrhea

- Commonly used PPIs (-prazole suffix):

  - Dexlansoprazole (Dexilant®)

  - Esomeprazole (Nexium®)

  - Lansoprazole (Prevacid®)

  - Omeprazole (Prilosec®)

  - Pantoprazole (Protonix®)

  - Rabeprazole (Aciphex®)

Other miscellaneous GI medications

These GI medications don't necessarily fit into another subcategory but are commonly used. The list below contains the generic and brand names with the usual indication for each drug.

- Hyoscyamine (Levsin®) – anticholinergic / antispasmodic

- Linaclotide (Linzess®) – irritable bowel syndrome (IBS) with constipation

- Lubiprostone (Amitiza®) – chronic constipation

- Naloxegol (Movantik®) – opioid-induced constipation

- Plecanatide (Trulance®) – IBS with constipation

- Ursodiol (Actigall®) – gallstone solubilizing agent

3: Endocrine system medications

Diabetes medication

The indications for diabetes medication are prediabetes, type 1 diabetes mellitus (T1DM), and type 2 diabetes mellitus (T2DM).

A T1DM patient requires multiple insulin injections daily (or an insulin pump) since their pancreas produces little to zero insulin. A patient with T2DM is usually prescribed at least one glucose-lowering medication. Insulin might be added to the regimen if blood glucose is not well-controlled. T2DM is much more common than T1DM in the U.S., mainly due to the prevalence of obesity.

Below are the different types of diabetes medication.

Insulin

- Indications: can be used for both T1DM and T2DM (insulin stimulates the uptake of glucose into cells from the blood)

- Adverse drug reactions: pain or irritation at injection site, hypoglycemia (low blood sugar)

- Commonly used insulins (insulins are categorized by their onset and duration of action):

Type of insulin	Onset of action	Duration of action	Examples
Rapid-acting insulin	5–20 minutes	3–5 hours	Insulin aspart (Novolog®), insulin glulisine (Apidra®), insulin lispro (Humalog®)

Short-acting insulin	30 mins	6–10 hours	Regular human insulin (Humulin R®, Novolin R®) (no Rx required)
Intermediate-acting insulin	1–2 hours	14–20 hours	Insulin NPH (Humulin N®, Novolin N®) (no Rx required)
Long-acting insulin	1–3 hours	18–24 hours	Insulin glargine (Basaglar®, Lantus®, Toujeo®), insulin detemir (Levemir®)
Ultra-long-acting insulin	2 hours	42 hours	Insulin degludec (Tresiba®)

Note: keep all insulin refrigerated until dispensed. Most insulin pens are stable at room temperature for 28 days. Certain long-acting insulins are stable at room temperature for longer (42 days for Levemir® and Toujeo®; 56 days for Tresiba®). The beyond-use date of most insulin vials is 28 days after the initial puncture of the rubber topper. Do not freeze insulin!

Biguanides

- Indications: prediabetes, T2DM

- Works in three ways:

  - Decreases the absorption of glucose

  - Improves the body's response to insulin

- Adverse drug reactions: diarrhea, nausea and vomiting, lactic acidosis

- Metformin is the only drug in the biguanide drug class. It is the most commonly prescribed glucose-lowering medication, and is available in two forms:

  - Metformin (Glucophage®)

- Metformin extended-release (Glucophage XR®, Fortamet®, others)

Note: the extended-release formulation of metformin has fewer GI side effects, but is more expensive than the immediate-release version.

Sulfonylureas

- Indication: T2DM (by stimulating insulin secretion)
- Adverse drug reactions: hypoglycemia, weight gain
- Commonly used sulfonylureas:

    - Glimepiride (Amaryl®)
    - Glipizide (Glucotrol®)
    - Glyburide (DiaBeta®)

Dipeptidyl peptidase-4 (DPP-4) inhibitors

- Indication: T2DM (by increasing insulin secretion and reducing glucagon release)
- Adverse drug reactions: hypoglycemia, joint pain, Steven-Johnson Syndrome (very rare)
- Commonly used DPP-4 inhibitors (-gliptin suffix):

    - Linagliptin (Tradjenta®)
    - Saxagliptin (Onglyza®)
    - Sitagliptin (Januvia®)

Glucagon-like peptide-1 (GLP-1) agonists

- Indication: T2DM (by increasing insulin release)
- Adverse drug reactions: diarrhea, nausea, vomiting, constipation
- Commonly used GLP-1 agonists (-glu/tide suffix):

- Exenatide (Byetta®)

- Exenatide extended-release (Bydureon®)

- Liraglutide (Victoza®)

- Dulaglutide (Trulicity®)

- Semaglutide (Ozempic®, Rybelsus®)

Note: GLP-1 agonists come as subcutaneous injections that must be stored refrigerated (except Rybelsus®, which is an oral tablet form of semaglutide).

Sodium-glucose transporter 2 (SGLT2) inhibitors

- Indication: T2DM (by increasing glucose elimination through the urine)

- Adverse drug reactions: urinary tract infections (UTIs), yeast infections

- Commonly used SGLT2 inhibitors (-gliflozin suffix):

  - Canagliflozin (Invokana®)

  - Dapagliflozin (Farxiga®)

  - Empagliflozin (Jardiance®)

  - Ertugliflozin (Steglatro®)

Hormone replacement therapy (HRT)

- Indications: hormone deficiency symptoms, development of secondary sex characteristics

  - For females, estrogen deficiency symptoms may include vaginal dryness and atrophy, insomnia, mood changes

  - For males, androgen deficiency symptoms may include reduced sex drive, hair loss, lean muscle loss, fatigue

- Adverse drug reactions: weight gain, mood changes, nausea, bloating

- Commonly used HRTs:

  - Estrogens and progestins:

    - Conjugated estrogen (Premarin®)

    - Conjugated estrogen-medroxyprogesterone (Prempro®)

    - Estradiol (Estrace®)

    - Estradiol-norethindrone (Activella®)

    - Micronized progesterone (Prometrium®)

  - Androgens (also known as anabolic steroids):

    - Testosterone cypionate (Depo-testosterone®)

    - Testosterone enanthate (Delatestryl®)

    - Testosterone gel (Androgel®, Testim®)

Thyroid hormone medications

Hypothyroidism medications

- Indication: hypothyroidism (underactive or surgically removed thyroid)

- Adverse drug reactions: weight loss, tremors

- Commonly used hypothyroidism medications:

  - Levothyroxine (Synthroid®)

  - Liothyronine (Cytomel®)

  - Thyroid desiccated (Armour Thyroid®)

Hyperthyroidism medications

- Indication: hyperthyroidism (overactive thyroid)

- Adverse drug reactions: sore throat, fever, unusual bleeding

- Commonly used hyperthyroidism medications:

  - Methimazole (Tapazole®)

  - Propylthiouracil (PTU®)

4: Immune system medications

Antibiotics

There are several classes of antibiotics. Each class of antibiotic has a different mechanism of action that targets different components of the bacteria – either to weaken or kill the bacteria.

- Indication: bacterial infections

- Adverse drug reactions: stomach upset, diarrhea (patients may take antibiotics with snacks or small meals to alleviate these symptoms)

- Commonly used antibiotics:

  - Amoxicillin (Amoxil®)

  - Amoxicillin/clavulanate (Augmentin®)

  - Azithromycin (Zithromax®, Z-pak®)

  - Sulfamethoxazole/Trimethoprim (Bactrim®)

  - Ciprofloxacin (Cipro®)

  - Levofloxacin (Levaquin®)

  - Metronidazole (Flagyl®)

  - Vancomycin (Vancocin®)

Note: it is important to finish taking a whole course of antibiotics to prevent antibiotic-resistant bacteria.

Antifungal agents

- Indication: fungal infections

- Adverse drug reactions: acid reflux, nausea, vomiting, skin burning, or irritation from topical formulations

- Commonly used antifungal agents:

  - Ketoconazole (Nizoral®)

  - Terbinafine (Lamisil®)

  - Micafungin (Mycamine®)

  - Griseofulvin (Gris-PEG®)

Antineoplastics (chemotherapy)

- Indication: cancer

- Adverse drug reactions: numerous and variable, but usually include nausea, vomiting, diarrhea, alopecia, fatigue, increased risk of infections

- Commonly used subtypes of antineoplastic drugs:

  - Alkylating agents:

    - Cyclophosphamide (Cytoxan®)

    - Temozolomide (Temodar®)

  - Platinum-based chemotherapy (-platin suffix):

    - Carboplatin (Paraplatin®)

    - Cisplatin (Platinol®)

    - Oxaliplatin (Eloxatin®)

  - Taxanes (-taxel suffix):

    - Docetaxel (Taxotere®)

- Paclitaxel (Taxol®)

- Pyrimidine antimetabolites:

    - 5-Fluorouracil (AKA 5-FU) (Adrucil®, Carac®, Efudex®)

    - Capecitabine (Xeloda®)

    - Gemcitabine (Gemzar®)

Antiviral agents

- Indications: viral infections such as herpes simplex, cytomegalovirus, herpes zoster, influenza prophylaxis, chickenpox, viral infection prophylaxis for organ transplant recipients

- Adverse drug reactions: headache, nausea, vomiting, diarrhea, constipation

- Commonly used antiviral agents:

    - Acyclovir (Zovirax®)

    - Amantadine extended-release (Gocovri®)

    - Famciclovir (Famvir®)

    - Oseltamivir (Tamiflu®)

    - Valacyclovir (Valtrex®)

Antiretroviral therapy (ART)

- Indication: human immunodeficiency virus (HIV) (by limiting the progression of HIV to AIDS)

- Adverse drug reactions: diarrhea, skin rash, nausea, vomiting, depression, liver damage

- There are multiple types of ARTs and they are often combined in one pill; here are a few of the most commonly used HIV medications:

- Abacavir/dolutegravir/lamivudine (Triumeq®)

- Efavirenz/emtricitabine/tenofovir (Atripla®)

- Etravirine (Intelence®)

- Emtricitabine/tenofovir (Truvada®)

- Lopinavir/ritonavir (Kaletra®)

Note: ARTs have multiple drug interactions, and patients should always consult their physicians or pharmacists before initiation of any new over-the-counter (OTC) or prescription medications.

Immunosuppressants

There are many types of immunosuppressants used in the treatment of numerous autoimmune disorders, immune system conditions, and certain cancers. The main adverse drug reaction for all immunosuppressants is an increased risk of infections. Below are some of the most common immunosuppressant drug names and their main indications.

General immunosuppressants

- Colchicine (Colcrys®, Mitigare®) – gout arthritis flares

- Methotrexate (Trexall®) – rheumatoid arthritis (RA), certain cancers

- Hydroxychloroquine (Plaquenil®) – lupus, RA

- Tacrolimus (Prograf®) – prevent rejection of transplanted organ

Biologics

Biologic drugs, sometimes called monoclonal antibodies, work in the immune system to reduce inflammation. They are used to treat numerous autoimmune conditions affecting the GI tract, skin, and joints. Some examples include RA, plaque psoriasis, ankylosing spondylitis, Crohn's disease, and ulcerative colitis. All of these products require refrigeration and some must be administered by a healthcare professional.

Some commonly prescribed biologics are:

- Adalimumab (Humira®)

- Etanercept (Enbrel®)

- Infliximab (Remicade®)

- Tofacitinib (Xeljanz®)

Steroids

- Indications: many autoimmune disorders, asthma, urticaria

- Adverse drug reactions:

  - ADRs with short-term use: insomnia, irritability, increased appetite

  - ADRs with long-term use: hypertension, hyperglycemia, edema, osteoporosis, cataracts, infections

- Commonly used steroids (-sone suffix for most steroids):

  - Dexamethasone (Decadron®)

  - Hydrocortisone (Cortef®)

  - Methylprednisolone (Solu-Medrol®, Medrol®)

  - Prednisolone (Orapred®, Prelone®, others)

  - Prednisone (Deltasone®, Sterapred®)

5: Musculoskeletal system medications

Bisphosphonates

- Indication: osteoporosis

- Adverse drug reactions: nausea, abdominal pain

- Commonly used bisphosphonates (-dron/ate/ic suffix):

    - Alendronate (Fosamax®)

    - Ibandronate (Boniva®)

    - Zoledronic acid (Zometa®)

Muscle relaxants

- Indication: muscle spasm

- Adverse drug reactions: drowsiness, dizziness, hypotension

- Commonly used muscle relaxants:

    - Carisoprodol (Soma®)

    - Cyclobenzaprine (Flexeril®)

    - Tizanidine (Zanaflex®)

6: Nervous system medications

Analgesics

Acetaminophen (APAP)

Acetaminophen is in its own medication class. It is available over-the-counter (OTC) as a generic product or as the brand Tylenol®. Acetaminophen is also an ingredient in many OTC and prescription combination products.

- Indications: pain, fever

- Adverse drug reactions: mild nausea, rare skin reactions, liver toxicity

Note: an overdose of acetaminophen can cause liver damage or death. For adults, the maximum daily dosage (MDD) of APAP is 3 to 4 grams (3,000 to 4,000 mg) per 24 hours. For pediatric patients, the weight-based dosing on the OTC product packaging should not be exceeded.

COX-2 inhibitors

- Indications: acute and chronic pain or inflammation, arthritis

- Adverse drug reactions: stomach upset, headache, drowsiness

- Commonly used COX-2 inhibitors:

  - Celecoxib (Celebrex®)

  - Meloxicam (Mobic®)

Narcotic analgesics

- Indication: acute and chronic pain that is unrelieved by other treatment types

- Adverse drug reactions: nausea, vomiting, constipation with chronic use, sedation, respiratory depression

- Commonly used narcotic analgesics:

  - Fentanyl (Duragesic®)

  - Hydrocodone/acetaminophen (Vicodin®)

  - Hydromorphone (Dilaudid®)

  - Methadone (Methadose®, Dolophine®)

  - Morphine (Roxanol®)

  - Oxycodone (OxyContin®)

- Oxycodone/acetaminophen (Percocet®)

Note 1: narcotic opioid analgesics are Schedule II controlled substances due to their high potential for abuse, misuse, and physical dependence.

Note 2: naloxone (Narcan®) is the antidote for opioid overdose.

Nonsteroidal anti-inflammatory drugs (NSAIDs)

- Indications: pain, fever, inflammation

- Adverse drug reactions: stomach ulcer or bleeding, heartburn, upset stomach, nausea, hypertension, drowsiness, rash, tinnitus

- Commonly used NSAIDs:

  - Diclofenac (Voltaren®)

  - Ibuprofen (Advil®, Motrin®)

  - Naproxen (Aleve®, Naprosyn®)

Salicylates

- Indications: pain, fever, inflammation

- Adverse drug reactions: stomach ulcer or bleeding, heartburn, upset stomach, nausea, hypertension, drowsiness, rash, tinnitus (i.e. similar to NSAIDs)

- Commonly used salicylates:

  - Aspirin

  - Magnesium salicylate (Nuprin)

Note 1: low-dose aspirin (81 mg) is also indicated for the prevention of cardiovascular events due to its blood-thinning effect.

Note 2: salicylates are not recommended for children or adolescents due to the risk of Reye's syndrome, which is a serious and sometimes fatal condition in pediatric patients.

Anesthetics

- Indications:

- Local anesthetics: to numb a select area before surgery or procedures (some are also used as analgesics or antiarrhythmics)

- General anesthetics: to induce sedation before surgery or procedure

- Adverse drug reactions:

  - ADRs for local anesthetics: blurred vision, headache, muscle twitching, prolonged numbness or weakness

  - ADRs for general anesthetics: confusion, short-term memory loss, dizziness, nausea, vomiting, shivering

- Commonly used anesthetics (-caine suffix for local anesthetics):

  - Bupivacaine (Marcaine®) – local anesthetic

  - Lidocaine (Xylocaine®) – local anesthetic

  - Propofol (Diprivan®) – general anesthetic

Anticonvulsants/anti-epileptic drugs (AEDs)

There are many types of epilepsy and dozens of different AEDs available; drug selection is individualized depending on the patient's age, child-bearing potential, and the type and severity of their seizures. While the primary indication is epilepsy, AEDs are also indicated for other neurological/mood disorders such as fibromyalgia and bipolar disorder.

- Adverse drug reactions: dizziness, drowsiness (varies with individual drug)

- Most commonly used AEDs:

- Cannabidiol (Epidiolex®)

- Carbamazepine (Tegretol®)

- Gabapentin (Neurontin®)

- Oxcarbazepine (Trileptal®)

- Phenytoin (Dilantin®)

- Lamotrigine (Lamictal®)

- Levetiracetam (Keppra®)

- Topiramate (Topamax®)

- Valproic acid (Depakote®)

Antidepressants

There are several types of antidepressants, which have different indications and adverse drug reactions. Here are some of the most common:

Selective serotonin reuptake inhibitors (SSRIs):

- Indications: depression, anxiety, eating disorders
- Adverse drug reactions: nausea, diarrhea, serotonin syndrome, bodyweight fluctuation, sexual dysfunction
- Commonly used SSRIs (-pram suffix for some):
  - Citalopram (Celexa®)

  - Escitalopram (Lexapro®)

  - Fluoxetine (Prozac®)

  - Paroxetine (Paxil®)

  - Sertraline (Zoloft®)

Serotonin-norepinephrine reuptake inhibitors (SNRIs):

- Indications: depression, anxiety disorders, fibromyalgia, diabetic peripheral neuropathy, eating disorders

- Adverse drug reactions: nausea, diarrhea, serotonin syndrome, bodyweight fluctuation, cardiovascular effects (such as hypertension and heart palpitations)

- Commonly used SNRIs:

    - Duloxetine (Cymbalta®)

    - Desvenlafaxine (Pristiq®)

    - Venlafaxine (Effexor XR®)

    - Levomilnacipran (Fetzima®)

Tricyclic antidepressants (TCAs):

- Indications: depression, generalized eating disorders, diabetic peripheral neuropathy, migraine prevention

- Adverse drug reactions: dry mouth, weight gain, reduced libido, erectile dysfunction, tachycardia

- Commonly used TCAs:

    - Amitriptyline (Elavil®)

    - Doxepin (Sinequan®)

    - Imipramine (Tofranil®)

    - Nortriptyline (Pamelor®)

Benzodiazepines (BZDs)

- Indications: anxiety, agitation, alcohol withdrawal, seizures, insomnia

- Adverse drug reactions: drowsiness, dependence

- Commonly used BZDs (-azepam or -azolam suffix):

  - Alprazolam (Xanax®)

  - Clonazepam (Klonopin®)

  - Diazepam (Valium®)

  - Midazolam (Versed®)

  - Temazepam (Restoril®)

  - Triazolam (Halcion®)

Note 1: BZDs are Schedule IV controlled substances due to their mild potential for abuse and addiction.

Note 2: flumazenil (Romazicon®) is the antidote for BZD overdose.

Migraine treatments

- Indication: migraine headaches

- Adverse drug reactions: dizziness, chest discomfort

- Commonly used migraine treatments:

  - Selective 5-HT receptor agonists ("triptans"):

    - Sumatriptan (Imitrex®)

    - Rizatriptan (Maxalt®)

    - Zolmitriptan (Zomig®)

  - Calcitonin gene-related peptides (CGRPs) – injectable drugs that work to prevent recurrent migraine headaches:

    - Erenumab (Aimovig®)

    - Galcanezumab (Emgality®)

- Miscellaneous combination analgesics for migraines:
    - Acetaminophen-butalbital-caffeine (Fioricet®)
    - Aspirin-butalbital-caffeine (Fiorinal®)
    - Aspirin-acetaminophen-caffeine (Excedrin Migraine®)

Sedatives

- Indication: insomnia
- Adverse drug reactions: drowsiness, somnolence the next day
- Commonly used sedatives:
    - Eszopiclone (Lunesta®)
    - Zolpidem (Ambien®)

Note 1: these drugs may also have a risk of sleep-walking, sleep-driving, and other behaviors, followed by short-term memory loss of these events.

Note 2: all drugs in this class are Schedule IV controlled substances.

Stimulants

- Indications: attention deficit hyperactivity disorder (ADHD), narco-lepsy
- Adverse drug reactions: insomnia, hypertension, dependency
- Commonly used stimulants (which should be administered in the morning to avoid insomnia):
    - Amphetamine/dextroamphetamine (Adderall®)
    - Atomoxetine (Strattera®)
    - Lisdexamfetamine (Vyvanse®)
    - Methylphenidate (Ritalin®)

- Methylphenidate ER (Concerta®, Daytrana®, others)

Note: all stimulants are Schedule II controlled substances (except atomoxetine).

7: Ophthalmic system medications

Beta-blockers (ophthalmic)

- Indication: glaucoma

- Adverse drug reactions: hypotension, bradycardia

- Commonly used ophthalmic beta-blockers:

    - Timolol (Timoptic®)

    - Betaxolol (Betoptic S®)

Prostaglandin analogs

- Indication: glaucoma

- Adverse drug reactions: dry eye, blurred vision, iris discoloration, eye inflammation, eyelash growth

- Commonly used prostaglandin analogs:

    - Bimatoprost (Lumigan®)

    - Latanoprost (Xalatan®)

    - Travoprost (Travatan®)

Note: bimatoprost is also marketed under the brand name Latisse® – a product that is indicated for eyelash growth.

8: Reproductive system medications

Oral contraceptives

- Indication: prevent pregnancy

- Adverse drug reactions: increased risk for stroke, depression, breast tenderness

- Commonly used oral contraceptives:

  - Ethinyl estradiol/desogestrel (Cyclessa®, Kavira®)

  - Ethinyl estradiol/drospirenone (Yasmin®, Yaz®)

  - Ethinyl estradiol/etonogestrel (Nuvaring®)

  - Ethinyl estradiol/norethindrone (Loestrin Fe®)

Note: many medications can interact with oral contraceptives, so patients must consult their doctors or pharmacists before initiation.

Phosphodiesterase type 5 inhibitors (PDE-5 inhibitors)

- Indication: male erectile dysfunction

- Adverse drug reactions: headache, flushing, priapism

- Commonly used PDE-5 inhibitors:

  - Sildenafil (Viagra®)

  - Tadalafil (Cialis®)

Note: PDE-5 inhibitors can cause severe hypotension when co-administered with nitrates. This drug interaction can result in death and the combination is contraindicated.

Selective estrogen receptor modulators (SERMs)

- Indications: fertility treatment, breast cancer, osteoporosis

- Adverse drug reactions: hot flashes, flu-like symptoms

- Commonly used SERMs:

    - Clomiphene (Clomid®)

    - Raloxifene (Evista®)

    - Tamoxifen (Nolvadex®)

9: Respiratory system medications

Antihistamines

- Indication: allergies (e.g. dust mite allergy, pollen allergy)

- Adverse drug reactions: drowsiness (first generation), dry mouth

- Commonly used first-generation antihistamine:

    - Diphenhydramine (Benadryl®)

- Commonly used second-generation antihistamines:

    - Cetirizine (Zyrtec®)

    - Fexofenadine (Allegra®)

    - Levocetirizine (Xyzal®)

    - Loratadine (Claritin®)

Antitussives

- Indication: acute cough

- Adverse drug reactions: headache, dizziness, nausea, stomach upset

- Commonly used antitussives:

- Benzonatate (Tessalon Perles®)

- Dextromethorphan (Delsym® and an ingredient in numerous other Rx and OTC products)

Decongestants

- Indications: nasal or sinus congestion

- Adverse drug reactions: loss of appetite, insomnia, hypertension, tachycardia, hyperactivity (especially in children)

- Commonly used decongestants:

  - Phenylephrine (Sudafed PE®)

  - Pseudoephedrine (Sudafed®)

Inhaled beta-agonists

- Indications: asthma, COPD

- Adverse drug reactions: tachycardia, palpitations

- Commonly used inhaled beta-agonists (-erol suffix):

  - Albuterol (ProAir®, Ventolin®, Proventil HFA®) – short-acting

  - Levalbuterol (Xopenex HFA®) – short-acting

  - Formoterol (Foradil Aerolizer®) – long-acting

  - Salmeterol (Serevent®; salmeterol is also an ingredient in other combination inhalers such as Advair®) – long-acting

Inhaled anticholinergics

- Indication: COPD

- Adverse drug reactions: constipation, dry mouth

- Commonly used anticholinergics (-tropium suffix):

- Ipratropium (Atrovent®)

- Tiotropium (Spiriva® Respimat or HandiHaler)

Inhaled/nasal corticosteroids

- Indications: asthma, COPD

- Adverse drug reactions: upper respiratory tract infection, oral thrush (to avoid oral thrush, patients must rinse mouth after each use)

- Commonly used inhaled corticosteroids:

    - Mometasone (Asmanex®, Nasonex®)

    - Fluticasone (Flovent®, Flonase®)

    - Budesonide (Pulmicort®, Rhinocort®)

    - Beclomethasone (Qvar RediHaler®, Beconase®)

Leukotriene modifiers

- Indications: asthma, allergies

- Adverse drug reactions: diarrhea, fever, headache, cold-like symptoms, depression/suicidal behaviors (rarely)

- Commonly used leukotriene modifiers (-lukast suffix):

    - Montelukast (Singulair®)

    - Zafirlukast (Accolate®)

Other miscellaneous respiratory medications

These respiratory medications don't fit into a subcategory above but are commonly used. The list below contains the generic and brand names with the usual indication for each drug.

- Cromolyn sodium (Gastrocrom®, Nasalcrom®) – mastocytosis

- Guaifenesin (Mucinex®, Robitussin®, others) – expectorant (works by increasing the water content of airway secretions, making mucus easier to expectorate)

- Theophylline (Theo-24®) – asthma and COPD

10: Urinary system medications

Alpha-blockers

- Indications: hypertension, benign prostatic hypertrophy (BPH)

- Adverse drug reactions: headache, dizziness, orthostatic hypotension

- Commonly used alpha-blockers (-osin suffix):

  - Alfuzosin (Uroxatral®)

  - Doxazosin (Cardura®)

  - Prazosin (Minipress®)

  - Tamsulosin (Flomax®)

Anticholinergic/antimuscarinic drugs for overactive bladder (OAB)

- Indication: relieves symptoms of OAB including urinary urgency, frequency, and incontinence

- Adverse drug reactions: dry mouth, blurred vision, constipation

- Commonly used anticholinergics for OAB:

  - Darifenacin (Enablex®)

  - Oxybutynin (Ditropan XL®, Oxytrol®)

  - Solifenacin (Vesicare®)

  - Tolterodine (Detrol LA®)

Other miscellaneous urinary system drugs

Here is a list of other common urinary system generic medications along with their brand names and main indication:

- Mirabegron (Myrbetriq®) – indicated for overactive bladder

- Potassium citrate (Urocit-K®) – urinary alkalinizer to treat and prevent certain types of kidney stones

- Phenazopyridine (Azo Urinary Pain Relief®, Pyridium®) – relieves UTI symptoms

Note: phenazopyridine turns urine bright orange, can discolor other bodily fluids, and may stain contact lenses.

Fixed-combination prescription drugs

Fixed-combination drug products contain more than one active ingredient. These may contain two or more drugs from the same or different class of medications. Combination products can improve patient adherence by reducing the number of medications or injections they need to take per day. Fixed-combination products may also be developed to minimize the potential for abuse of the main active ingredient.

The generic drug names for fixed-combination products are usually separated by a forward slash. Some examples include:

- Amlodipine/atorvastatin (Caduet®) – a combination of a CCB with a statin in one tablet, indicated for patients with both hypertension and hypercholesterolemia.

- Amlodipine/valsartan/hydrochlorothiazide (Exforge HCT®) – similar to Caduet®, but this product contains valsartan instead of atorvastatin and also includes a diuretic for added control of hypertension; a total of three active ingredients in one tablet.

- Insulin glargine/lixisenatide injection (Soliqua®) – a combination of a long-acting insulin with a GLP-1 receptor agonist in one injection, indicated for type 2 diabetes mellitus.

- Diphenoxylate/atropine (Lomotil®) – this fixed-combination anti-diarrheal product is a controlled substance due to the diphenoxylate ingredient, but its combination with atropine decreases its potential for misuse.

Vitamins

There are 13 essential vitamins required for the body to work properly. Vitamins are grouped into two categories: fat-soluble and water-soluble.

Fat-soluble vitamins are stored in the body's fatty tissue. These include A, D, E, and K.

- Vitamin A: retinol – important for vision health

- Vitamin D: D2 (ergocalciferol); D3 (cholecalciferol) – aids nerve and immune function, aids in calcium absorption

- Vitamin E: alpha-tocopherol – antioxidant properties

- Vitamin K: phytonadione – blood clot formation

Water-soluble vitamins are not stored in large amounts by the body. The body absorbs the water-soluble vitamins it needs from the diet (or vitamin supplements), and any leftover amounts are flushed out through the urine.

- Vitamin B1: thiamine – metabolizes carbohydrates

- Vitamin B2: riboflavin – metabolizes fats, protein, and carbohydrates

- Vitamin B3: niacin – manages cholesterol and triglyceride levels

- Vitamin B5: pantothenic acid – helps convert nutrients into energy

- Vitamin B6: pyridoxine – aids immune system, commonly used for morning sickness

- Vitamin B7: biotin – metabolizes nutrients, thought to strengthen hair/skin/nails

- Vitamin B9: folate – cell development, routinely used in pregnancy

- Vitamin B12: cobalamin – aids red blood cell production, nerve cell function

- Vitamin C: ascorbic acid – antioxidant and immune system functions, aids iron absorption and cartilage formation

Practice Questions: Medications

Answers and explanations can be found at the end of the questions.

Question 1: Ortho Tri-Cyclen® and Tri-Sprintec® are approved by the FDA to be therapeutically equivalent. Which of the following statements is incorrect?

    a)   They are pharmaceutically equivalent

    b)   They produce almost identical clinical effect(s)

    c)   They are proven to have the same safety profile

    d)   They have the same appearance

Question 2: St. John's Wort can cause a serious interaction with which of the following medications?

    a)   Amlodipine

    b)   Duloxetine

    c)   Lisinopril

    d)   Verapamil

Question 3: Which one of the following drugs does not require therapeutic monitoring to ensure patient safety and therapeutic level?

    a)   Phenytoin

    b)   Tacrolimus

    c)   Eszopiclone

    d)   Rifampin

Question 4: Mrs. Smith was diagnosed with an upper respiratory infection three days ago. Her primary care physician prescribed her medications for this condition. Today, she checked her blood glucose as directed for her diabetes. The glucose reading is higher than usual. Which of the following medications can cause a rise in her blood glucose?

a)   Azithromycin

b)   Benzonatate

c)   Prednisone

d)   Oxymetazoline

Question 5: On 05/01/2020, a Humalog® vial was opened to make a patient-specific insulin drip. What is the beyond-use-date (BUD) of this vial after it was opened and punctured?

a)   Six hours after the initial puncture

b)   05/08/2020

c)   05/10/2020

d)   05/29/2020

Question 6: What is the mechanism of action of Imitrex®?

a)   5-HT receptor agonist

b)   Monoamine oxidase inhibitor

c)   Serotonin and norepinephrine inhibitor

d)   GABA agonist

Question 7: A patient drops off a prescription for carbamazepine. The prescription calls for carbamazepine suspension 200 mg PO TID x 30 days. The pharmacy has one 450 mL bottle of carbamazepine oral suspension with a concentration of 100 mg/5 mL. Would this one bottle of carbamazepine be sufficient to fill this prescription?

a)   Yes. The required volume to fill this prescription is 150 mL

b) Yes. The required volume to fill this prescription is 450 mL

c) No. The required volume to fill this prescription is 900 mL

d) No. The required volume to fill this prescription is 180 mL

Question 8: Concurrent use of nitroglycerin with _____ is absolutely contraindicated.

a) Sildenafil

b) Sumatriptan

c) Furosemide

d) Ketorolac

Question 9: _____ must be protected from light.

a) IV levofloxacin

b) IV vancomycin

c) IV gentamicin

d) IV ceftriaxone

Question 10: Which of the following medications should not be split or crushed?

a) Depakote® ER

b) Coreg®

c) Novasc®

d) OxyContin®

Answers and Explanations: Medications

Question 1: answer d) They have the same appearance

Two medications are deemed to be therapeutically equivalent when they are pharmaceutically equivalent, and when they also have the same or almost identical clinical effect and safety profile. Two drugs have to be pharmaceutically equivalent first, before they can be therapeutically equivalent.

Two medications are proven to be pharmaceutically equivalent if they:

- Contain the same chemical entity

- Contain the same quantity of active ingredient

- Have the same dosage form

- Have the same route of administration

Two therapeutically equivalent medications might have differences of appearance: shape, scoring, release mechanism, coloring, packaging, flavoring.

Question 2: answer b) Duloxetine

St. John's Wort can cause serious side effects when being co-administered with a selective serotonin-reuptake (SSRI) such as duloxetine. It can result in the accumulation of serotonin that leads to serotonin syndrome. Serotonin syndrome is presented with flu-like symptoms such as fever, shivering, and fever.

Question 3: answer c) Eszopiclone

Phenytoin is an anti-epileptic drug. Tacrolimus is an immunosuppressant to prevent organ rejection in renal and liver transplant. Eszopiclone is the generic name for Lunesta®, treating insomnia. Rifampin is an antimycobacterial used with other medications to treat tuberculosis.

Phenytoin, tacrolimus, and rifampin are some of the narrow therapeutic index (NTI) drugs, where a very small change in dosing can result in significant therapeutic outcome(s). NTIs require frequent pharmacokinetics and pharmacodynamics therapeutic monitoring to ensure a patient's safety and treatment success.

Question 4: answer c) Prednisone

A diagnosis of bacterial upper respiratory tract infection is typically treated with an antibiotic such as azithromycin (a macrolide) and a corticosteroid like prednisone, along with other therapies to alleviate symptoms. Benzonatate is used to relieve cough, while oxymetazoline (Afrin®) is a nasal decongestant that should only be used for a short period of time due to potential rebound congestion.

Prednisone is an anti-inflammatory agent that helps by reducing the inflammation of the airway. As with any other corticosteroids, prednisone can cause a spike in blood glucose by making the liver resistant to insulin.

Question 5: answer d) 05/29/2020

Multi-dose insulin vials such as Humalog® can be stored at room temperature for 28 days after initial entry.

Question 6: answer a) 5-HT receptor agonist

Imitrex® is the brand name of sumatriptan. Sumatriptan is one of the "-triptans" drugs that are used to treat migraine symptoms. Sumatriptan exerts its effects by binding to 5-HT receptors, causing constriction of cerebral blood vessels which alleviate painful symptoms of migraine.

Question 7: answer c) No. The required volume to fill this prescription is 900 mL

The amount of carbamazepine (in mg) needed to fill this prescription:

200mg x 3 x 30 = 18,000 mg

Using the available stock bottle with the 100mg / 5mL concentration, the volume needed to fill this prescription is: 100 mg / 5 mL = 18,000 mg / x

x = (18,000 mg x 5 mL) / 100 mg = 900 mL

Question 8: answer a) Sildenafil

Nitroglycerin is a nitrate. Sildenafil (Viagra®) is a phosphodiesterase-5 inhibitor. Both of these drug classes cause smooth muscle relaxation that result in a drop of blood pressure. Co-administration of these two medications can cause severe hypotension and even death.

Question 9: answer a) IV levofloxacin

IV levofloxacin needs to be protected from light to maintain the medication's integrity. The oral formulation of levofloxacin is not sensitive to light. Ceftriaxone vials should be protected from light, but after reconstitution into intravenous solution, protection from light is not necessary.

Question 10: answer a) Depakote® ER

Generally, controlled-release or extended-release medications should not be crushed or split: it may compromise the release mechanism of the medication. Follow each product's labeled guidance from the drug manufacturer.

Knowledge Domain 2:
Federal
Requirements

Acts and Amendments
You Should Know

Laws and regulations govern virtually every aspect of pharmacy. As a pharmacy technician, it's important to have a basic understanding of federal laws and how they protect patients.

Pure Food and Drug Act (1906)

- Prohibits interstate commerce of misbranded and adulterated drugs and foods.

- This legislation was spurred by shockingly unsanitary conditions in the meat-packing industry, exposed by Upton Sinclair's *The Jungle.*

- Definitions to know:

- Misbranded: a drug product is misbranded if its labeling is inaccurate, incomplete, or misleading.

- Adulterated: a drug product that fails to meet quality, strength, or purity standards.

Federal Food, Drug, and Cosmetic Act (1938)

- Requires drug manufacturers to provide the FDA with evidence of safety by submitting a New Drug Application before marketing them.

- This act essentially created the FDA and started a new system of drug regulation.

- If the FDA does not take any action within 60 days, the drug is automatically approved. (Note: the Kefauver-Harris Amendment of 1962 invalidated this aspect of the Act.)

Durham-Humphrey Amendment (1951)

- Defines two specific categories for drug products: legend drugs (prescription-only) and over-the-counter (OTC) medication.

- Legend drug labels must indicate "Caution: Federal law prohibits dispensing without a prescription."

Kefauver-Harris Amendment (1962)

- Established a framework that requires drug manufacturers to scientifically prove that a medication is not only safe but effective.

- Prior to this amendment, drug manufacturers only had to prove that a drug was safe (not misbranded or adulterated).

Note: the FDA's automatic 60-day approval time frame (see Federal Food, Drug, and Cosmetic Act above) became invalid with this amendment.

Controlled Substances Act (CSA) (1970)

The Controlled Substances Act is the federal drug policy that regulates the manufacture, importation, possession, use, and distribution of controlled substances: certain narcotics, stimulants, depressants, hallucinogens, and anabolic steroids.

The CSA classifies controlled substances into five schedules represented by Roman numerals: Schedules I, II, III, IV, and V. The abbreviation "C" followed by a Roman numeral is the designation found on controlled substance product labels.

Drugs are placed into their respective schedules based on their medical use and potential for abuse or dependence.

CSA classifications

Schedule I controlled substances (C-I)

- C-I drugs have a high potential for abuse and physical/psychological dependence.

- They currently have no accepted medical use and are considered investigational or illicit drugs.

- Examples include heroin, methaqualone, and marijuana. (Note: marijuana is considered a Schedule I drug at the federal level by the DEA even though it is legalized for medical or recreational use in many states.)

Schedule II controlled substances (C-II)

- C-II drugs have a high potential for abuse and physical/psychological dependence. However, unlike C-I drugs, C-II drugs are considered medically acceptable and necessary.

- The CSA sets forth more strict regulations on the prescribing, distribution, and dispensing of C-II controlled substances in comparison to CIII–V.

- Examples include most narcotics and stimulants.

- Narcotic examples: codeine (single ingredient), morphine, oxycodone

- Stimulant examples: amphetamine, methylphenidate

Schedule III controlled substances (C-III)

- C-III drugs have moderate to low potential for physical dependence but a high potential for psychological dependence.

- Examples include anabolic steroids, buprenorphine, and certain codeine fixed-combination products.

Schedule IV controlled substances (C-IV)

- C-IV drugs have a low potential for abuse and dependence. However, C-IV drugs could still lead to addiction and have dangerous effects, especially if combined with other substances of abuse.

- Examples include benzodiazepines (e.g. alprazolam), some muscle relaxants (e.g. carisoprodol), tramadol, and zolpidem.

Schedule V controlled substances (C-V)

- C-V drugs have a low potential for abuse and dependence. These products may contain limited quantities of certain narcotics.

- Examples include antidiarrheals (e.g. atropine/diphenoxylate) and antitussives (e.g. guaifenesin/codeine).

The Drug Enforcement Agency (DEA) implements the CSA and may prosecute violators of these laws. Anyone who orders, handles, stores, and distributes controlled substances must be registered with the DEA to perform these tasks. (Exception: registration is waived for any official of the U.S. Army, Navy, Marine Corps, Air Force, Public Health Services, or Bureau of Prison.)

Important aspects of the CSA

Before you read the most important/relevant aspects of the CSA below, please be aware of the following information:

- The term "written" is used interchangeably with "issued" regardless of the method used to communicate the prescription to the pharmacy (verbally telephoned, faxed, electronic, or handwritten on paper).

- Prescriptions for non-controlled substances expire one year after the date written.

- When federal and state laws are different, pharmacies are expected to follow the more stringent law.

- Over the past two decades, modernization amendments have been made to the CSA due to advancements in technology. These details can be accessed in the Code of Federal Regulations Title 21. Some of these latest updates are included below.

Controlled substance (CS) prescription refills

- C-II: refills not permitted. A new prescription must be issued for each fill.

  However, prescribers can issue three 30-day supply prescriptions to create a 90-day supply for their patients with an established diagnosis. In such situations, the date of issuance for all three supplies must be the same, and there must be a "Do not fill until/before" date on the second and third prescriptions.

  Example: a patient drops off three 30-day-supply prescriptions for Adderall® – each of which was written on 01/01/2021. The issuance date on all three should be 01/01/2021. The second prescription states "Do not fill until 01/31/2021," and the third prescription states "Do not fill until 03/02/2021." The second and third prescriptions may not be filled before the date noted, but they may be filled on or after the date noted.

- C-III–IV: prescriptions can have up to five refills or refills for up to six months from the date of issuance – whichever comes first.

- C-V: can be refilled as many times as authorized by prescriber per federal law, but state laws may differ.

CS prescription expiration

- C-II: no expiration per federal law, but may have an expiration date per state law or company policy.

- C-III–IV: valid for six months from the date of issuance.

- C-V: no expiration per federal law, but may have an expiration date per state law or company policy.

CS prescription partial fills

- C-II: partial fill is permitted as long as the remainder is filled within 72 hours. If the remainder is not filled within 72 hours, the remainder is void, and the prescriber must be notified.

- C-III–V: partial fills are permitted with no time limit – as long as the prescription is not expired (i.e. six months from the written date).

Transferring CS prescription for refill

- C-II: transfer prohibited.

- C-III–V: allow one-time transfer between two pharmacies. Pharmacies electronically sharing a real-time, online database may transfer up to the maximum refills permitted by the law and by the prescriber.

Maintenance of CS records

- C-II: records must be stored separately from all other prescription records.

- C-III–V: records must be stored separately from other prescription records or marked in the lower right corner with the letter "C" in red ink, at least one inch high. (Then they can be stored in the same file with non-controlled substance prescription records.)

- Note: these recordkeeping rules apply to hardcopy prescriptions only. Electronic prescriptions may be stored in a readily retrievable electronic database.

Maintenance of CS inventory

- Initial inventory: when issued a DEA registration, a pharmacy must take an initial inventory (an actual physical count of all controlled substances in their possession) and record this information.

- Biennial inventory: DEA registrants are required to take a new CS inventory at least every two years.

- C-II: CS inventory records must be filed separately from C-III–V CS inventory records. These records are not sent to the DEA but must be kept on file for at least two years.

- C-I: CS products must be stored in a secure, lockable "substantially constructed cabinet" (usually a safe or vault).

- C-II–V: CS products must be stored in a secure, lockable "substantially constructed cabinet" (usually a safe or vault) OR may be dispersed throughout the stock of non-controlled substances in such a manner that deters theft or diversion.

Distributing or receiving CS inventory

- C-II: may use DEA Form 222 (a physical paper form) to document receiving or distributing C-II products into or out of inventory. Executed forms must be kept on file for at least two years.

- Note: the DEA Controlled Substance Ordering System (CSOS) allows secure electronic ordering of C-II controlled substances without an accompanying DEA Order Form 222.

- C-III–V: all transactions can be recorded using invoices.

Disposal of CS inventory

- On-site disposal of controlled substances must be in the presence of a DEA agent or authorized personnel.

- When utilizing a reverse distributor, the transaction must be documented on a DEA Form 222. A reverse distributor is a processor that receives expired or unwanted CS inventory from a DEA registrant and returns it to the manufacturer or arranges for its disposal.

- For returns or manufacturer recalls, CS must be delivered to the source where it was purchased. This transaction must be documented on a DEA Form 222.

Required information for CS prescription

- Patient's full name and address

- Prescriber's name, address, and DEA number

- Drug name, strength, and dosage form

- Quantity prescribed

- Date issued

- Direction for use

- Prescriber's signature

Note: A prescriber must physically sign a paper prescription as they would any other legal document. Signature stamps or computer-generated signatures are not permitted. A computer-generated CS prescription that is printed out or faxed by the prescriber must be manually signed.

DEA forms

- DEA Form 41: for reporting the destruction of CS

- DEA Form 104: for reporting pharmacy closure or surrender of a pharmacy permit

- DEA Form 106: for reporting loss or theft of CS

- DEA Form 222: for ordering C-I and C-II CS

- DEA Form 222a: for ordering more of Form DEA 222

- DEA Form 224: for applying for a DEA registration number

- DEA Form 224a: for a DEA registration renewal; must be renewed every three years

Be familiar with DEA Form 222

The original DEA Form 222 is a triplicate form. It consists of three layers of paper printed with different colored inks with carbon paper in between. The carbon automatically copies what is written on the top layer to all three layers. The triplicate DEA Form 222 is being phased out, and will no longer be accepted after October 30, 2021, but this information may still appear on the exam.

- The first page, the original (brown ink): must be retained by the CS supplier.

- The second page, copy 2 (green ink): CS supplier sends this page to the DEA.

- The third page, copy 3 (blue ink): pharmacy retains this page for at least two years.

In September 2019, the DEA implemented a new single-sheet official DEA Form 222.

- The purchaser must make a copy of the original single-sheet DEA Form 222 and submit the original to the supplier. The copy may be kept in electronic or paper form.

- The supplier must provide a copy of each original single-sheet DEA Form 222 to the DEA. The copy may be mailed or emailed by the close of the month during which the order is filled.

DEA number verification

A prescriber cannot legally prescribe a CS unless they are registered with the DEA. The prescriber must include their DEA number on the face of all CS prescriptions (or provide their DEA number over the phone if it is missing or if the prescription is verbally issued).

DEA numbers have two letters followed by seven numbers. The first letter identifies the type of practitioner:

- A, B, and F: physicians, dentists, veterinarians, pharmacies, and hospitals

- M: allied health ("mid-level") practitioners such as physician assistants and nurse practitioners

- P and R: manufacturers, distributors, narcotic treatment programs, and researchers

The second letter represents the first letter of the prescriber's last name or the first letter of the business name of a hospital or pharmacy.

There are four steps to verify a DEA number:

1. Add the 1st, 3rd, and 5th digits of the DEA number.
2. Add the 2nd, 4th, and 6th digits of the DEA number, then multiply this sum by 2.
3. Add the results from Step 1 and Step 2 together.
4. The sum from Step 3 will be a two-digit number. The second digit of this two-digit number will match the 7th (the final) digit of the DEA number.

Exemptions: officials of the US Air Force, Army, Navy, Marines, and Public Health Services are not required to register with the DEA to prescribe CS.

Poison Prevention Packaging Act (PPPA) (1970)

- Aims to protect young children from poisonings and deaths that can occur if they gain access to hazardous products including medications.

- Requires that most over-the-counter and legend drugs be packaged in child-resistant containers. Some products are exempt from the PPPA, such as sublingual nitroglycerin, effervescent acetaminophen, effervescent aspirin, oral contraceptives, and hormone replacement therapy.

- Requires that child-resistant packaging be designed to make it significantly difficult for children under five years of age to open within a reasonable time, but not too difficult for the majority of the adult population.

- Note: child-resistant containers are not "childproof" – they simply delay the child's access to the content of the containers by a reasonable amount of time.

Federal Anti-Tampering Act (1983)

- Mandates that over-the-counter (OTC) drug products must have a tamper-evident seal.

- Sometimes called the "Tylenol Act." It was passed in response to the deaths of seven people who took Tylenol capsules that had been laced with cyanide in Chicago.

Prescription Drug Marketing Act (1987)

- Prohibits the selling, purchasing, and trading of prescription drug samples.

- Limits the distribution of drug samples only to those licensed to prescribe them, if requested.

Omnibus Budget Reconciliation Act (OBRA) (1990)

Commonly called "OBRA '90," this Act established three key pharmacy provisions: drug utilization review, patient counseling standards, and patient record maintenance.

Drug utilization review (DUR)

- Also known as drug or medication utilization evaluation (DUE or MUE), DUR requires pharmacists to review if the prescription is necessary and appropriate. There are two types of DUR: prospective and retrospective.

- Prospective DUR is performed by a pharmacist before a drug is dispensed and considers the following factors:

- Therapeutic duplications – are multiple drugs prescribed from the same drug class or for the same indication?

- Drug interactions – are there any interactions (such as drug-drug or drug-disease interactions)?

- Drug allergies – has the patient had past allergic reactions to any medications?

- Over/underutilization – is the dosage and duration of treatment appropriate?

- Potential misuse – are there patterns or signs of drug abuse or misuse?

- Retrospective DUR is performed after the patient has received the medication and is often used to detect prescribing or dispensing patterns.

Patient counseling standards

- An offer to counsel must be made to every patient.

- Counseling information may include drug name, its intended use and expected action, route of administration, dosage, common side effects including their avoidance and mitigation, proper storage, potential interactions, and action to be taken in the event of a missed dose.

- Note 1: states have formed their own regulations in response to OBRA '90 and patient counseling requirements vary from state to state. However, in all states, pharmacy technicians should always direct patient counseling questions to a pharmacist – even if they know the answer.

- Note 2: be sure to remember that counseling is defined as the act of providing pertinent drug information to a patient by a pharmacist.

Patient record maintenance

- Patient records, often called patient profiles, should be accurately maintained by all pharmacy staff.

- Keep the following information updated in patient profiles: full name, date of birth (DOB), address, phone numbers, gender, drug allergies, chronic conditions, insurance information, and complete record of medications.

Originally, OBRA '90 was geared to reduce federal spending by requiring these pharmacy services for Medicaid recipients (disabled or low-income individuals who receive government assistance). The end result of the legislation was that these services were provided to *all* patients, not just Medicaid recipients.

Dietary Supplement Health and Education Act (DSHEA) (1994)

- Under this act, dietary supplements such as vitamins and herbal supplements are considered "food." Therefore, dietary supplements do not have to be approved or authorized for investigation as a new drug by the FDA.

Health Insurance Portability and Accountability Act (HIPAA) (1996)

- Limits the use and disclosure of protected health information (PHI) to the "minimum necessary."

- Provides an option for the patient to obtain a copy of their health record and request corrections.

- If PHI is exposed to unauthorized parties, the affected individuals must be notified.

Food and Drug Administration Modernization Act (FDAMA) (1997)

- This act eliminates certain labeling requirements. For example, the statement "Caution: Federal law prohibits dispensing without a prescription" may be stated as "Rx only."

Drug Addiction Treatment Act (DATA) (2000)

- Allows qualified prescribers to complete training and register for a NADEAN (Narcotic Addiction DEA Number).

- A NADEAN (a special DEA number that begins with the letter "X") enables them to prescribe Schedule III, IV, and V controlled substances indicated for the treatment of opioid use disorder (OUD) outside of an addiction treatment center.

- Note: buprenorphine is the most commonly prescribed medication for OUD. Prescriptions issued for buprenorphine-containing products must include the prescriber's NADEAN and DEA number to be considered valid.

Combat Methamphetamine Epidemic Act (CMEA) (2005)

- Regulates the sale of over-the-counter products containing pseudoephedrine (PSE) and ephedrine, which can be used to illegally manufacture methamphetamine ("meth"). These products must be stored behind the counter or in a locked cabinet.

- Requires that customers present a valid, government-issued photo ID to purchase PSE-containing products.

- Customer purchase limits for OTC products:

- Daily limit: 3.6 grams/day per customer

- No more than 9 grams per 30 days if purchased in-store

- No more than 7.5 grams per 30 days if purchased via mail order or mobile retail vendor (such as an airport kiosk)

- Pharmacies must keep a written or electronic record of all OTC sales of PSE and ephedrine products. The records must be maintained for at least two years and include the following:

- Product name and quantity sold

- Name, address, and signature of the purchaser

- Date and date of the sale

- As part of CMEA, annual certification is required for all sellers of PSE and ephedrine products. The certification confirms that the seller has trained all of their employees and is compliant with these regulations.

Practice Questions: Federal Requirements

Answers and explanations can be found at the end of the questions.

Question 1: A prescription label states "glipizide 5 mg tablet, take 1 tablet by mouth every day with breakfast; #30". The prescription bottle contains 30 tablets of glyburide 5 mg. If the label satisfies all of the federal and state requirements, this prescription label is considered _____.

a) Adulterated

b) Misbranded

c) Adulterated and misbranded

d) Appropriate, since it was transcribed correctly from the doctor's order

Question 2: DEA Form 222 must be maintained and made available for inspection for _____.

a) 12 months

b) 2 years

c) 3 years

d) 5 years

Question 3: Which of the following medications is not required to be dispensed in a child-resistant container?

a) Hydrocodone/acetaminophen

b) Sublingual nitroglycerin

c)   Ketorolac

d)   Zolpidem

Question 4: A patient drops off a prescription for 30 Vyvanse® 30 mg capsules. The pharmacy only has 15 capsules in stock. The patient accepts the partial fill of 15 capsules. The pharmacist shall provide the patient with the remaining 15 capsules within _____.

a)   24 hours

b)   72 hours

c)   7 days

d)   10 days

Question 5: The safety data sheet (SDS) is overseen by which of the following organizations?

a)   FDA

b)   OSHA

c)   BOP

d)   DEA

Answers and Explanations: Federal Requirements

Question 1: answer c) Adulterated and misbranded

According to the Food, Drug, and Cosmetic Act:

Adulteration occurs when the product has been mixed or packed with any substance which reduces its strength or quality, or the drug has been substituted in whole or in part, or the drugs are recognized in an official compendium but differ in strength, quality or purity. The bottle is supposed to contain 30 tablets of glipizide 5 mg, but instead it contains 30 tablets of glyburide 5 mg – which is an adulteration.

A drug is misbranded if the labeling is false and misleading; the label indicates that there are 30 tablets of glipizide 5 mg, when in fact there are 30 tablets of glyburide 5 mg – which is false and misleading.

This prescription is, therefore, both adulterated and misbranded.

Question 2: answer b) 2 years

According to the DEA, DEA Form 222 must be maintained separately from all other records of the registrant. DEA Form 222 is required to be kept available for inspection for a period of two years.

Question 3: answer b) Sublingual nitroglycerin

The Poison Prevention Packaging Act (PPPA) of 1970 requires that most over-the-counter products and legend drugs be packaged in child-resistant containers. Some of the products that are exempt from PPPA include:

sublingual nitroglycerin, effervescent acetaminophen, effervescent aspirin, oral contraceptives, and hormone replacement therapy.

Question 4: answer b) 72 hours

According to the DEA, a partial fill of a Schedule II drug is permissible if the pharmacist is not able to provide the whole amount written for in the prescription.

The remaining portion of the prescription may be filled within 72 hours of the first partial filling; however, if the remaining portion cannot be filled within the 72-hour period, the pharmacist shall notify the prescriber. No further quantity may be supplied beyond 72 hours without a new prescription.

Question 5: answer b) OSHA

The SDS, formerly known as MSDS (Material Safety Data Sheet) is overseen by the Occupational Safety and Health Administration (OSHA). The SDS includes information such as the properties of each chemical; the physical, health, and environmental health hazards; protective measures; and safety precautions for handling, storing, and transporting the chemical.

Knowledge Domain 3:
Patient Safety and Quality Assurance

Error Prevention

A strong focus on patient safety helps to protect patients from errors that could have detrimental consequences. Some definitions to know are:

- Medication error: any preventable event that may lead to inappropriate medication use or patient harm.

- Adverse drug event (ADE): harm experienced by a patient that results from exposure to a medication.

Note: not all medication errors lead to adverse drug events. Errors that are caught before they can result in injury are "near misses."

The Institute for Safe Medication Practices (ISMP) is a non-profit organization devoted entirely to error prevention and is known as the gold standard for medication safety. The following ISMP recommendations are proven to reduce medication errors.

Use tall-man lettering

This is the use of mixed-letter cases to emphasize the difference in drug names that look alike or sound like. For example:

- BuPROpion/BusPIRone

- HydrALAZINE/HydrOXYzine

- PredniSONE/PrednisoLONE

Use a leading zero

Omitting the leading zero can cause patients to receive doses that are much higher than intended. For example:

- Do use "0.5 g"

- Don't use ".5 g" as this can be mistaken for 5 g if the decimal point is not seen

Avoid a trailing zero

Using a trailing zero can cause patients to receive doses that are much higher than intended. For example:

- Do use "5 g"

- Don't use "5.0 g" as this can be mistaken for 50 g if the decimal point is not seen

Avoid error-prone abbreviations

The use of abbreviations can cause medication errors if they are misinterpreted, especially if handwritten. ISMP provides a list of error-prone abbreviations and The Joint Commission (TJC) designates certain abbreviations on its "Do Not Use" list. TJC is the accreditation group that develops patient safety and care standards for hospitals and other healthcare facilities.

Examples of error-prone abbreviations include:

- IU (international units) can be mistaken for IV (intravenous). Write "units" instead.

- QD or Q.D. (every day) can be mistaken for QID (4 times daily). Write "every day" or "daily" instead.

- MgSO4 (magnesium sulfate) can be mistaken for morphine sulfate. Write out full drug names.

- SS (one-half) can be mistaken for 55 (fifty-five). Write out "one half" or use "0.5."

Verbal order read back

Certified pharmacy technicians in certain states can receive verbal prescriptions for non-controlled drugs via telephone. Technicians must always reduce the order to writing, then read back to the prescriber to ensure the accuracy of the order. Keep in mind that this authority is only applicable in certain states.

Barcode and QR code scanning

- Barcode and QR code scanning can be used in both community and hospital pharmacies to reduce dispensing errors.

- Barcodes include the product's NDC (national drug code) number. NDCs are unique three-segment numbers that identify a drug product in the following format: XXXXX-XXXX-XX.

- The first segment of numbers identifies the drug manufacturer.

- The second segment of numbers identifies the drug.

- The third segment of numbers identifies the package size.

- QR codes include the NDC and also the product lot number and expiration date.

E-prescribing

- The e-prescribing (electronic) method can help to reduce errors that might occur from misinterpreting handwritten prescriptions.

- E-prescribing reduces the number of lost paper prescriptions.

- It speeds up the process of insurance verification and saves paper, time, and physical storage space.

The "7 rights" of medication administration

Medication errors occur when human factors lead to the inappropriate use of medications. The most common human factors are:

- Distractions – lapses in judgment when interrupted or multi-tasking

- Omissions – an ordered dose of a medication is not administered

All pharmacy and healthcare workers must make patient safety their top focus. This ensures the "7 rights" of medication administration:

1. Right patient
2. Right medication
3. Right dose
4. Right route
5. Right time
6. Right indication
7. Right documentation

Risk Evaluation and Mitigation Strategies (REMS)

A REMS program is a drug safety program that the FDA can require for manufacturers of certain medications. It places strict criteria and procedures on the prescribing and dispensing of specific medications that have serious safety concerns. REMS programs are unique for each drug, but usually require prescriber and patient registration and consent to monitoring such as blood testing. The most commonly prescribed drugs with REMS programs include:

- The clozapine REMS program helps to reduce the risk of severe neutropenia with this psychiatric drug.

- The iPLEDGE REMS program helps to reduce the risk of severe birth defects with isotretinoin – an anti-acne drug.

Beers Criteria for Potentially Inappropriate Medication Use in Older Adults

- The American Geriatrics Society (AGS) establishes and oversees the Beers Criteria for Potentially Inappropriate Medication Use in Older Adults – known as "Beers Criteria" or "Beers List."

- Beers medications have been associated with poor outcomes for older patients – such as confusion, falls, and mortality.

- When pharmacists receive warnings for Beers Criteria medications, prescribers should be contacted to discuss if the therapy is appropriate or if alternative therapies would be safer.

- Some of the drug classes (and examples) listed in Beers Criteria by the AGS are:

- First-generation antihistamines (diphenhydramine)

- Antiparkinson agents, e.g. bromocriptine

- Antithrombotics, e.g. clopidogrel (Plavix®)

- Anti-infective, e.g. nitrofurantoin (Macrobid®)

- Alpha-1 blockers, e.g. terazosin (Hytrin®)

- Benzodiazepines, e.g. alprazolam (Xanax®)

- Hypnotics, e.g. zolpidem (Ambien®)

- NSAIDs, e.g. ibuprofen (Advil®)

- Tricyclic antidepressants, e.g. nortriptyline (Pamelor®)

- Skeletal muscle relaxants, e.g. cyclobenzaprine (Flexeril®)

Pharmacy Technician Task Examples

The following lists are generalizations and do not include all job requirements. Refer to your state's pharmacy technician protocol as determined by your state's BOP (board of pharmacy).

Tasks you'll be expected to perform

- Create, maintain, and update patient profiles

- Receive written, faxed, and electronic prescriptions

- Perform prescription input

- Fill prescription orders including counting, packaging, and labeling

- Alert pharmacist about situations that require professional judgment

- Manage, restock inventory, and remove expired products from inventory

- Dispose of expired products per the organization's policy and procedures

- Maintain the order and cleanliness of the pharmacy

- Follow procedures to ensure the security of the prescription area

- Operate cash register

Tasks that must be performed by a pharmacist

- Drug utilization review (DUR)

- Therapeutic substitution

- Patient counseling – including over-the-counter (OTC) product recommendations

- Final verification of prescriptions

Event Reporting

MedWatch

A voluntary program established by the FDA to report adverse events or sentinel events that are observed in human medical products.

FDA Adverse Event Reporting Systems (FAERS)

A database that contains information on adverse event and medication error reports submitted to the FDA. These reports are received from healthcare professionals and consumers.

Vaccine Adverse Event Reporting System (VAERS)

Similar to FAERS and co-sponsored by the FDA and CDC, this program is used to collect and analyze data from adverse events after vaccination. The goal is to identify new safety concerns that were not discovered during clinical trials.

MEDMARX

An anonymous, online error-reporting program designed for hospitals and health systems. The United States Pharmacopeia (USP) oversees this program.

Hygiene and Cleaning Standards

What you should know

- Counting trays should be cleaned once daily with 70% isopropyl alcohol.

- Medication storage areas, including refrigerators, cannot contain food or drinks.

- Contaminated crash carts must be disinfected.

- Countertops must be cleaned daily with 70% isopropyl alcohol.

- Shelves, floors, and storage areas must be cleaned routinely and free of clutter.

Practice Questions:
Patient Safety and Quality Assurance

Answers and explanations can be found at the end of the questions.

Question 1: What is the appropriate way to write "four grams of magnesium sulfate" on a prescription?

a) 4 g of MS

b) 4.0 g of MS

c) 4 g of magnesium sulfate

d) 4.0 g of magnesium sulfate

Question 2: _____ is a post-marketing safety surveillance program that collects information about adverse events that occur after the administration of vaccination.

a) VAERS

b) FAERS

c) VIS

d) VAR

Question 3: While compounding sterile preparations, sterile gloves should be disinfected with _____.

a) 70% isopropyl alcohol (IPA)

b) Sterile water for injection

c) 0.9% sodium chloride

d) Hydrogen peroxide

Question 4: Which of the following statements about drug utilization evaluation (DUE) is not true?

a)   DUE is formerly known as DUR (drug utilization review)

b)   OBRA-90 mandates DUE

c)   DUE is mandated for the high-risk patient population only

d)   Drug interaction, allergy, and contraindication are among other components that must be evaluated during a DUE

Question 5: A prescription is written for Augmentin® 30mg/kg/day BID for 7 days for a 35 lbs pediatric patient. The pharmacy has Augmentin® 400 mg/5 mL in stock. What is the total volume required of the medication?

a)   20.8 mL

b)   41.7 mL

c)   45 mL

d)   60 mL

Question 6: A prescription is called in for Mr. Smith for Bactrim® 40–200 mg/5 mL with the direction to take 1 tsp PO BID x 10 days. Two ounces of the medication is dispensed to Mr. Smith. How many days of therapy will Mr. Smith be short?

a)   2 days

b)   3 days

c)   4 days

d)   5 days

Question 7: Mrs. Brown is on chronic opioid therapy for severe osteoarthritis. She experiences constipation after seven days of therapy. Constipation is considered a(n) _____.

a)   Adverse drug reaction

b) Side effect

c) Clinical misuse

d) Allergy

Question 8: Oral liquid phenytoin is ordered for a patient. The order is written for phenytoin 5mg/kg per day, divided in two doses. Duration of therapy is 10 days. Patient weighs 175 lbs. Pharmacy has one 8 oz bottle of phenytoin 125mg/5mL. How much volume is left in the bottle after dispensing the entire 10-day therapy for this patient?

a) 40 mL

b) 81 mL

c) 160 mL

d) One 8 oz bottle is not enough to dispense the entire 10-day therapy

Question 9: _____ is the process of comparing a patient's medication orders with all of the medication the patient had been taking as an outpatient.

a) Prospective drug utilization evaluation

b) Retrospective drug utilization evaluation

c) Medication reconciliation

d) Prior authorization

Answers and Explanations: Patient Safety and Quality Assurance

Question 1: answer c) 4 g of magnesium sulfate

Using a trailing zero or missing a leading zero could lead to error in the amount of drug due to the decimal point being ineligible or overlooked. A trailing zero is any zero that occurs after a decimal point, while a leading zero is any zero that occurs before the decimal point.

For example, ".5 g" is "0.5 g" expressed without the leading zero; the amount can be mistaken to be 5 g. On the other hand, "5.0 g" is "5 g" expressed with a trailing zero. "5.0 g" may be mistaken for "50 g" for the same reason regarding the decimal point.

Morphine sulfate or magnesium sulfate must not be abbreviated as "MS". "MS" can be mistaken for magnesium sulfate or morphine sulfate, so the drug names must be spelled out instead.

Question 2: answer a) VAERS

VAERS stands for Vaccine Adverse Event Reporting System, and it is co-sponsored by the FDA and the CDC. This program is used to collect and analyze data from adverse events after vaccination. The goal is to identify new safety concerns that were not discovered during clinical trials.

Question 3: answer a) 70% isopropyl alcohol (IPA)

Gloved hands can be disinfected by rubbing 70% IPA to all contact surfaces of the gloves and letting it dry completely. Routine application of sterile 70%

IPA is recommended throughout the compounding process and whenever non-sterile surfaces such as counter tops, chairs, and carts are touched.

Question 4: answer c) DUE is mandated for the high-risk patient population only

The Omnibus Budget Reconciliation Act of 1990 (OBRA-90) mandates drug utilization evaluation (formerly known as drug utilization review) on all new prescriptions. During this process, the new prescription is evaluated for drug interactions, drug-disease interactions, contraindication, and patient allergy.

Question 5: answer b) 41.7 mL

35 lbs = 35 / 2.2 = 15.9 kg

Total dispensed drug for 7 days: 30 mg/kg x 15.9 kg x 7 days = 3,339 mg

Total dispensed volume: 400mg/5mL = 3,339 mg / x

x = (3,339 mg x 5 mL) / 400 mg = 41.7 mL

Question 6: answer c) 4 days

The prescription requires: 5 mL x 2 x 10 = 100 mL of Bactrim®

Total dispensed volume: 2 oz x 30mL/oz = 60 mL

Difference: 100 mL - 60 mL = 40 mL

One day of therapy requires: 5mL x 2 = 10 mL

Patient will be short: 40 mL / 10 (mL/day) = 4 days

Question 7: answer b) side effect

Side effects may occur regardless of the dose. Because side effects are predictable the majority of the time, patients are counseled on it by physicians and pharmacists, so they know what to expect and how to handle them if they occur. Adverse drug reactions, on the other hand, can be predictable or unpredictable.

Question 8: answer b) 81 mL

175 lbs / 2.2 lbs/kg = 79.5 kg

Total 10-day therapy requires: 5mg/kg x 79.5 kg x 10 = 3,975 mg

Total volume needed for the 10 days of therapy: 125mg/5mL = 3,975 mg / x

X = 159 mL

8 oz = 240 mL

Volume left in the bottle: 240 mL - 159 mL = 81 mL

Question 9: answer c) Medication reconciliation

Medication reconciliation is the process of comparing a patient's inpatient medication orders with all of the outpatient medications. The purpose of medication reconciliation is to avoid/prevent medication duplication, omission, and drug interactions.

Knowledge Domain 4:

Order Entry and Processing

Non-Sterile Compounding

Extemporaneous compounding is the on-demand preparation of a drug product according to a physician's prescription, formula, or recipe in the event that the product is not commercially available or if there is a drug shortage.

Compounding often requires simple math calculations to determine the amount of ingredients needed. See the "Calculations Using Percentages" chapter for some practice questions and explanations. .

USP <795> provides guidance on good compounding practices in preparing non-sterile compounded drug products. These practices include:

- Rotate stock to ensure that the oldest stock gets used first.

- Prevent contamination when storing and handling ingredients and preparations.

- Equipment must be located in a way that makes it easy to use, maintain, and clean.

- Equipment cleaning must be performed immediately after compounding to prevent cross-contamination of the next batch preparation.

- The Class A balance should be used for all weighing required in prescription compounding. It has a minimum sensitivity of 6 milligrams (mg) and a maximum capacity of 120 grams (g). It may be an analog (torsion balance scale) or digital scale (preferred).

- The beyond-use date (BUD) is the date after which a compounded medication should not be used. Note, however, that the expiration date and BUD are not the same:

- Expiration dates are assigned by manufacturers.

- BUDs are assigned to compounded and repackaged products based on the institution's policy.

- Maximum beyond-use date for non-sterile compounded products:

- Non-aqueous (no water): 6 months

- Topical/dermal preparation that contains water: 30 days

- Oral formulations that contain water: 14 days (refrigerated)

- Non-sterile compounding techniques:

  - Spatulation: mixing powders and semi-solids (ointments, creams, etc.) on an ointment slab using a spatula. Involves no particle size reduction, so the powders must already be fine and of a uniform size.

  - Trituration: reducing the particle size of a substance by grinding using a mortar and pestle.

  - Levigation: decreasing the surface tension between two ingredients by wetting with a small amount of insoluble liquid (e.g. glycerin for oil-soluble bases and mineral oil for water-soluble bases), then spatulating or triturating.

Measurement Systems

- The apothecary system is, for the most part, outdated. Note that some of the very old drugs still have "grains" as their unit for strength.

- The avoirdupois system is the traditional system of weights and measures in the United States. It is based on pounds (lbs) and ounces (oz).

- The metric system is the standard measurement system around the world due to its accuracy and simplicity.

Note: you should know how to convert a patient's weight from pounds to kilograms when calculating weight-based dosing. See the "Calculations Using Conversions" chapter for some practice questions and explanations.

Conversions

Weight

- 1 milligram (mg) = 1,000 micrograms (mcg)

- 1 gram (g) = 1,000 milligrams (mg)

- 1 kilogram (kg) = 1,000 grams (g)

- 1 kg = 2.2 lbs

To convert a patient's weight from lbs to kg, divide weight in lbs by 2.2. For example: the patient weighs 189 lbs. 189/2.2 = 85.9 kg.

Volume

- 1 milliliter (mL) = 1 cm3 (cc)

- 1 deciliter (dL) = 100 mL

- 1 liter (L) = 1,000 mL

- 1 ounce (oz) = 30 mL

- 1 tablespoonful = 15 mL

- 1 teaspoonful = 5 mL

Roman numerals

- I = 1

- II = 2

- III = 3

- IV = 4

- V = 5

- VI = 6

- VII = 7

- VIII = 8

- IX = 9

- X = 10

- L = 50

- C = 100

- D = 500

- M = 1,000

Interpreting Prescription Sigs

Route of administration

- PO: by mouth

- PR: rectally

- AU: both ears

- AS: left ear

- AD: right ear

- OU: both eyes

- OS: left eye

- OD: right eye

- IV: intravenous

- IVPB: intravenous piggyback

- IM: intramuscular

- ID: intradermal

- NG: nasogastric

- SC or SQ: subcutaneous

- SL: sublingual

- TD: transdermal

Dosing frequencies

- QD: daily

- QOD: every other day

- BID: twice daily

- TID: three times daily

- QID: four times daily

- QAM: every morning

- QPM: every evening

- Qwk: every week

- HS: bedtime

- AC: before meals

- PC: after meals

- PRN: as needed

- STAT: immediately

Calculations Using Conversions

As a pharmacy technician, you'll need to use your knowledge and basic math skills to solve pharmacy calculations. Next, we'll cover some common examples of dosage calculations.

The following dosage chart shows the recommended dosage of amoxicillin, adapted from the drug's prescribing information. This chart will help you answer the sample questions below.

Type of infection	Severity	Usual dosage for adults and children (weight ≥ 40 kg)	Usual dosage for children (age > 3 months)
Ear, nose, throat	Mild/moderate	500 mg every 12 hours	25 mg/kg/day in divided doses every 12 hours
	Severe	875 mg every 12 hours	45 mg/kg/day in divided doses every 12 hours

Sample question 1

Calculate the proper dosage of amoxicillin for Jane. She has a severe ear infection. She is seven years old and weighs 55 lbs. She has no known drug allergies. What is the correct dosage for Jane? (Hint: one kilogram is equal to 2.2 pounds.)

a)   500 mg every 12 hours

b)   562.5 mg every 12 hours

c)   625 mg every 12 hours

d)   1,125 mg every 12 hours

Correct answer: b) 562.5 mg every 12 hours

Explanation:

To solve this problem, the first step is to convert the patient's weight in pounds (lbs) to kilograms (kg). Remember: 1 kilogram = 2.2 lbs. So, divide the patient's weight by 2.2:

$$55 \div 2.2 = 25 \text{ kg}$$

Next, we look at the dosage chart. It indicates that the dosage for a severe ear infection for Jane's age and weight is 45 mg/kg/day in divided doses every 12 hours. So, multiply the patient's weight by 45 mg/kg:

$$45 \text{ mg/kg/day} \times 25 \text{ kg} = 1,125 \text{ mg/day}$$

Now we know that the total dosage is 1,125 mg per day. But according to the chart, this must be divided every 12 hours. If a drug is given every 12 hours, we know the patient will get 2 doses per day. So, divide the total dosage by 2:

$$1,125 \text{ mg} \div 2 = 562.5 \text{ mg}$$

Sample question 2

The pediatrician ordered amoxicillin 400 mg/5 mL suspension for Jane. Using the dosage calculated above, what is the volume (mL) that Jane should receive for each dose?

a) 5 mL

b) 7 mL

c) 14 mL

d) 112.5 mL

Correct answer: b) 7 mL

Explanation:

First, we organize the information we already know and identify our "X" (what we're trying to solve for):

We know that the amoxicillin ordered is 400 mg/5 mL.

We know Jane needs 562.5 mg per dose.

We need to calculate X mL that Jane will receive for each dose.

We calculate this by setting up a simple proportion, then cross-multiply:

$$\frac{400 \text{ mg}}{5 \text{ mL}} = \frac{562.5 \text{ mg}}{X \text{ mL}}$$

(400 mg) × (X mL) = (562.5 mg) × (5 mL) ... which equals:

$$(400) \times (X \text{ mL}) = 2{,}812.5$$

Then, divide both sides by 400 to solve for X:

$$\frac{(400) \times (X \text{ mL})}{400} = \frac{2{,}812.5}{400}$$

Or, written another way:

2,812.5 ÷ 400 = 7.03 mL ... for practical purposes, we'll round this to 7 mL.

Sample question 3

You check your inventory and see that the pharmacy only has amoxicillin 250 mg/5 mL suspension in stock. Using the information above, what is the total volume of medication that Jane will require for a 10-day course?

    a)   11 mL

    b)   110 mL

    c)   140 mL

    d)   225 mL

Correct answer: d) 225 mL

Explanation:

To calculate this answer, you have to recognize that you need the dosage you calculated from sample question 1 (562.5 mg). Then, set up a proportion and cross-multiply as in sample question 2:

$$\frac{250 \text{ mg}}{5 \text{ mL}} = \frac{562.5 \text{ mg}}{X \text{ mL}}$$

(250 mg) × (X mL) = (562.5 mg) × (5 mL) ... which equals:

(250) × (X mL) = 2,812.5

Then, divide both sides by 250 to solve for X:

$$\frac{(250) \times (X \text{ mL})}{250} = \frac{2{,}812.5}{250}$$

Or, written another way:

$$2{,}812.5 \div 250 = 11.25 \text{ mL}$$

Now that we've calculated the volume needed for one dose, we can multiply by the total doses per day to get the total volume per day:

$$11.25 \text{ mL} \times 2 \text{ doses per day} = 22.5 \text{ mL total per day}$$

Last, we multiply the total volume per day by the total number of days of therapy to get the answer:

$$22.5 \text{ mL total per day} \times 10 \text{ days} = 225 \text{ mL total volume required}$$

Note: this answer (225 mL) is the correct answer. However, most antibiotic suspensions come in certain sizes of bottled powder for reconstitution. For example, amoxicillin suspension may come in 100 mL and 150 mL bottles.

So, the pharmacy staff would reconstitute and dispense the number of bottles that satisfy the total required volume. The pharmacy staff would advise the patient's parents to discard the leftover suspension after the 10-day course is completed.

Calculations Using Percentages

Pharmacy technicians should know how to calculate the amount of active ingredients needed to compound a product with a percentage strength. **The main concept to remember is this: percentages always refer to units per 100 total units.** This applies to units of weight (grams) and units of volume (milliliters) as follows:

%W/W (percent weight/weight)

This is used when the active drug and the inactive base are both in the same unit of weight: grams (g).

By definition, 1% = 1 g of active ingredient per 100 g of total product. (1% = 1g/100g).

%V/V (percent volume/volume)

This is used when the active drug and the inactive base are both in the same unit of volume: milliliters (mL).

By definition, 1% = 1 mL of active ingredient per 100 mL of total product. (1% = 1mL/100mL).

%W/V (percent weight/volume)

This is used when the active drug is in the unit of weight, grams, and the inactive base is in the unit of volume, milliliters.

By definition, 1% = 1g of active ingredient per 100 mL of total product (1% = 1g/100 mL).

Sample question

You are working in a community compounding pharmacy. You're asked to prepare 80 grams of a 10% hydrocortisone cream. How much hydrocortisone powder do you need?

a)   0.8 g

b)   8 g

c)   10 g

d)   80 g

Correct answer: b) 8 g

Explanation:

To calculate the amount of hydrocortisone powder needed, set up a proportion. A 10% cream contains 10 grams per 100 grams. But since we want to determine the amount needed in 80 grams, we would solve for X by cross-multiplying:

$$\frac{10\text{ g}}{100\text{ g}} = \frac{X\text{ g}}{80\text{ g}}$$

$(10 \text{ g}) \times (80 \text{ g}) = (100 \text{ g}) \times (X) \dots$ which equals:

$$(100) \times (X) = 800$$

Then, divide both sides by 100 to solve for X:

$$\frac{(100) \times (X)}{100} = \frac{800}{100}$$

… which equals: X = 8 g

If instead you were asked to calculate the amount of active ingredient needed to compound 80 mL of a 10% solution, the answer would be the same. The only difference is that instead of dividing by 100 grams, you would divide by 100 mL.

Practice Questions:
Order Entry and Processing

Answers and explanations can be found at the end of the questions.

Question 1: What does the DAW (dispense as written) Code 1 mean?

   a)   No production selection indicated

   b)   Substitution allowed by provider

   c)   Brand drug mandated by law

   d)   Substitution not allowed by provider

Question 2: What is the smallest volume of liquid that can be measured in a 50 mL cylinder?

   a)   3 mL

   b)   5 mL

   c)   10 mL

   d)   20 mL

Question 3: Which of the following information is required by the FDA on a prescription of Ambien®?

   a)   Prescriber's DEA number

   b)   Patient's date of birth

   c)   Patient's Medicaid number

   d)   Third party payor's group number

Question 4: A prescription is written for moxifloxacin ophthalmic solution. The sig is "2gtt tid ou x 10d". How many drops will the patient use in total?

a)   12 drops

b)   60 drops

c)   84 drops

d)   120 drops

Question 5: A prescription for Bactrim® 40–200/5 mL is written with the following sig: "1 tsp PO BID x 7d, then 1 tsp PO daily x 7d". How many oz of this medication should be dispensed?

a)   2.3 oz

b)   3.5 oz

c)   4.7 oz

d)   5.5 oz

Question 6: A six-year-old female patient received 3 L of normal saline in 24 hours. The standard infusion rate for pediatric patients is 75 mL/hr. How much excess normal saline in milliliters did the patient receive per hour?

a)   15 mL

b)   25 mL

c)   50 mL

d)   55 mL

Question 7: An order is written for gentamicin IV 125 mg in 100 mL 0.9% NaCl. Gentamicin is available in 80 mg/mL vial. How many millimeters of gentamicin are needed to compound this preparation?

a)   1.25 mL

b)   1.56 mL

c) 2.1 mL

d) 2.4 mL

Question 8: A physician calls in an order for 1 L of 5% iodine. The pharmacy has 3% iodine tincture and 8% iodine tincture in stock. How many mL of the 3% iodine tincture should be used?

a) 300 mL

b) 500 mL

c) 600 mL

d) 800 mL

Question 9: A patient has an order of levetiracetam 500 mg IV BID for his five-day hospitalization. The pharmacy has levetiracetam 500 mg/5 mL injection in stock. How many mL of the levetiracetam 500 mg/5 mL injection is needed to compound the IV preparation of levetiracetam for his whole hospital stay?

a) 10 mL

b) 20 mL

c) 40 mL

d) 50 mL

Answers and Explanations: Order Entry and Processing

Question 1: answer d) Substitution not allowed by provider

DAW stands for "dispense as written". DAW codes provide information to pharmacists regarding whether or not the prescribed medication can be substituted for another product. DAW Code 1 indicates that a substitution is not allowed by the provider.

DAW Code 0 means no product selection has been indicated (so it would allow pharmacists to dispense the generic version of the prescribed brand name medication – e.g. carvedilol can be dispensed in place of Coreg®).

Question 2: answer c) 10 mL

The amount of liquid to be measured in a graduated cylinder shall not be less than 20%.

Question 3: answer a) Prescriber's DEA number

Ambien® is a Schedule IV controlled substance. The prescriber's DEA number is required on all controlled substance prescriptions.

Question 4: answer d) 120 drops

[(2 drops x 3 times per day) x 2 eyes] x 10 days = 120 drops

Question 5: answer b) 3.5 oz

Use 30 mL for 1 fluid oz

(5 mL x 2 times per day x 7 days) + (5 mL x 7 days) = 105 mL

105 mL x (1oz / 30 mL) = 3.5 oz

Question 6: answer c) 50 mL

What patient received: 3,000 mL / 24 hr = 125 mL/hr

125 mL - 75 mL = 50 mL

Question 7: answer b) 1.56 mL

80 mg / 1 mL = 125 mg / x

X = 125 mg / 80 mg = 1.56 mL

Question 8: answer c) 600 mL

The goal of alligation is to compound a solution of desired concentration from two available solutions with different concentrations.

Step 1: determine the number of parts of the available solution with the lower concentration (3%) that will be needed to compound the desired solution (5%). This number of parts is equal to the differences between the higher concentration (8%) and the desired concentration (5%). The difference is 3 parts (8 - 5 = 3). Therefore, 3 parts of the 3% iodine solution will be needed.

Step 2: similar to step one. The number of parts of the higher concentration solution (8%) that will be needed is equal to the difference between the lower concentration (3%) and the desired concentration (5%), which is 2 (5 - 3 = 2). Therefore 2 parts of the 8% iodine solution will be needed.

Step 3: 1,000 mL is the desired volume (1 L = 1,000 mL) and it is divided into 5 parts: 2 parts 8% iodine solution and 3 parts 3% iodine solution.

Step 4: set up the ratio and determine the needed volume of the available solution.

1,000 mL / 5 parts = x mL (of 3% iodine solution) / 3 parts

X = (1,000 mL x 3 parts) / 5 parts

X = 600 mL of 3% iodine solution

In order to determine the volume of the 8% iodine solution that is needed, you can subtract the volume of 3% iodine solution from the desired volume of the 5% iodine solution:

1,000 mL - 600 mL = 400 mL of 8% iodine solution

Question 9: answer d) 50 mL

Total amount in mg of levetiracetam needed for the whole hospital stay: 500 mg x 2 x 5 days = 5,000 mg

500 mg / 5 mL = 5,000 mg / x mL

x = 50 mL

You're Done!

Congratulations on finishing *PTCB Hero: The Essential Information You Need to Pass the First Time (and Nothing Else!)*.

Do you want to cement your knowledge and make sure you *really* understand it? Do you wish to feel reassured that you can recall that knowledge under exam conditions – with the types of questions that will appear on the real thing?

Then look no further than **PTCB Hero Online** – the perfect complement to this book. **PTCB Hero Online** contains hundreds of practice questions PLUS two simulated exams (which replicate the real-life exams you'll be taking). All the practice questions and simulated exam questions include detailed explanations of the correct answers afterward.

When you buy **PTCB Hero Online**, you'll get:

- **Hundreds of practice questions** with complete explanations (focus on one knowledge domain at a time, or mix them up)

- **Two simulated exam**s with complete explanations

- **A condensed version of this book** – so you can learn on your device whenever you have a spare moment

PTCB Hero Online is compatible with computers, smartphones, and tablets, so you can access it whichever way you please.

Visit www.ptcbhero.co and enter 30OFFNOW at checkout for 30% off.

If you have any questions or concerns before you buy, simply email admin@medicalhero.co and we'll get back to you right away!

Good luck in your exam, and please do let us know how you do: contact us at admin@medicalhero.co and share your success story!

The Medical Hero Team

Made in the USA
Las Vegas, NV
21 September 2024

95575549R00103